Reflective Practice in Nursing

Sara Miller McCune founded SAGE Publishing in 1965 to support the dissemination of usable knowledge and educate a global community. SAGE publishes more than 1000 journals and over 800 new books each year, spanning a wide range of subject areas. Our growing selection of library products includes archives, data, case studies and video. SAGE remains majority owned by our founder and after her lifetime will become owned by a charitable trust that secures the company's continued independence.

Los Angeles | London | New Delhi | Singapore | Washington DC | Melbourne

4th Edition

Reflective Practice in Nursing

Philip Esterhuizen

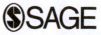

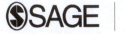

Learning Matters
An imprint of SAGE Publications Ltd
1 Oliver's Yard
55 City Road
London EC1Y 1SP

SAGE Publications Inc.
2455 Teller Road
Thousand Oaks, California 91320

SAGE Publications India Pvt Ltd
B 1/I 1 Mohan Cooperative Industrial Area
Mathura Road
New Delhi 110 044

SAGE Publications Asia-Pacific Pte Ltd
3 Church Street
#10-04 Samsung Hub
Singapore 049483

First edition published 2010
Second edition 2013
Third edition 2016
Fourth edition 2019

Editor: Donna Goddard
Development editor: Sarah Turpie
Senior project editor: Chris Marke
Project management: Swales & Willis Ltd, Exeter,
Devon
Marketing manager: George Kimble
Cover design: Wendy Scott
Typeset by: C&M Digitals (P) Ltd, Chennai, India
Printed in the UK

Library of Congress Control Number: 2019931374

British Library Cataloguing in Publication Data

A catalogue record for this book is available from the
British Library

ISBN 978-1-5264-6005-9
ISBN 978-1-5264-6006-6 (pbk)

At SAGE we take sustainability seriously. Most of our products are printed in the UK using responsibly sourced
papers and boards. When we print overseas we ensure sustainable papers are used as measured by the
PREPS grading system. We undertake an annual audit to monitor our sustainability.

Contents

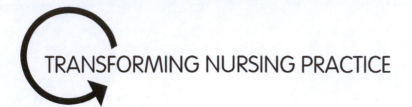

TRANSFORMING NURSING PRACTICE

Transforming Nursing Practice is a series tailor made for pre-registration students nurses. Each book in the series is:

 Affordable

 Full of active learning features

 Mapped to the NMC Standards of proficiency for registered nurses

 Focused on applying theory to practice

Each book addresses a core topic and they have been carefully developed to be simple to use, quick to read and written in clear language.

An invaluable series of books that explicitly relates to the NMC standards. Each book covers a different topic that students need to explore in order to develop into a qualified nurse... I would recommend this series to all Pre-Registered nursing students whatever their field or year of study.

LINDA ROBSON,
Senior Lecturer at Edge Hill University

Many titles in the series are on our recommended reading list and for good reason - the content is up to date and easy to read. These are the books that actually get used beyond training and into your nursing career.

EMMA LYDON,
Adult Student Nursing

ABOUT THE SERIES EDITORS

DR MOOI STANDING is an Independent Nursing Consultant (UK and International) and is responsible for the core knowledge, adult nursing and personal and professional learning skills titles. She is an experienced NMC Quality Assurance Reviewer of educational programmes and a Professional Regulator Panellist on the NMC Practice Committee. Mooi is also Board member of Special Olympics Malaysia, enabling people with intellectual disabilities to participate in sports and athletics nationally and internationally.

DR SANDRA WALKER is a Clinical Academic in Mental Health working between Southern Health Trust and the University of Southampton and responsible for the mental health nursing titles. She is a Qualified Mental Health Nurse with a wide range of clinical experience spanning more than 25 years.

BESTSELLING TEXTBOOKS

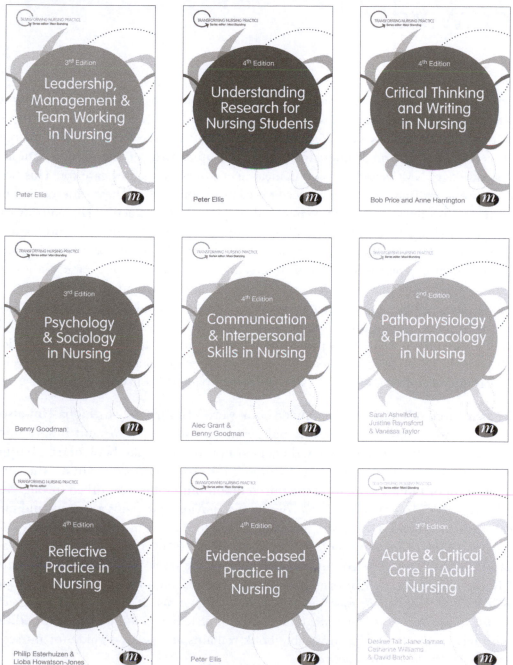

You can find a full list of textbooks in the
Transforming Nursing Practice series at
https://uk.sagepub.com

Foreword

The Transforming Nursing Practice series includes several titles that focus on developing nurses' personal and professional learning skills. *Reflective Practice in Nursing* is a great example in this respect. Lifelong learning in nursing involves a constant dialogue between nurses' personal inner world and the outer world of scientific, technological knowledge, NMC standards and clinical needs of patients they care for. This book carefully and skilfully shows the reader how to incorporate all of these different strands within their professional identity as nurses through reflective practice. High-quality care links personal attributes, like the ability to empathise with patients, with professional expertise in delivering thoughtful, relevant, person-centred evidence-based nursing interventions. Each chapter is loaded with interesting practical examples, case studies and learning activities to engage readers in reflecting on and developing their self-awareness, problem-solving skills and nursing knowledge that is grounded in interactions with service users. After reading this book, both nursing students and registered nurses will be well informed in applying the principles of reflective practice to review their interactions with patients. In doing so, readers will enhance their personal and professional development as nurses and their effectiveness in addressing patients' concerns.

The first three editions of this popular book were written solely by Lioba Howatson-Jones and were based on her original research into reflective and biographical learning. Lioba has since retired and decided not to update the book herself but graciously agreed to Philip Esterhuizen's offer to do so. The fourth edition therefore retains most of Lioba's work from the third edition but Philip has worked through and updated each chapter to ensure *Reflective Practice in Nursing* remains a current and practical guide for nurses. The most significant change to the fourth edition is the adoption of the *Standards of Proficiency for Registered Nurses* (NMC, 2018a) which are linked to each chapter in the book. The continuing relevance of the book is supported by the latest NMC standards under 'Platform 1: Being an accountable professional' which states, *Registered nurses continually reflect on their practice and keep abreast of new and emerging developments in nursing, health and care* (NMC, 2018a, p8). In updating the fourth edition Philip has ensured that this invaluable book remains an essential guide for nurses to reflect and develop their practice.

Dr Mooi Standing

Series Editor

Acknowledgements

This book reflects 40 years of nursing, teaching and research experience. I would, therefore, like to dedicate the work to the countless patients, colleagues, students and research participants who have allowed me to develop my knowledge and understanding, and to reflect on my personal and professional development and insights.

My acknowledgement to those who have inspired me along my professional and personal journey would be incomplete without a personal word of thanks to Professor Dawn Freshwater, Professor Christopher Johns, Dr Jean Watson and Professor Dagfinn Nåden. Each, in his or her own way – both personally and professionally – has taught me to embrace the courage needed to 'be' and embody reflection.

Thanks also to Dr Mooi Standing for her helpful suggestions in the editing of the chapters. I would also like to thank the editors at Sage.

Publisher's acknowledgements

We would like to acknowledge the hard work of Dr Lioba Howatson-Jones in first conceiving and writing this text for Learning Matters. Over the course of various editions this work has helped many students to understand the importance of reflection in their practice and to develop their reflective skills, and we are grateful that this text can continue to help students for many editions to come.

About the authors

Dr Philip Esterhuizen is a Lecturer in the School of Healthcare at the University of Leeds where he teaches undergraduate and postgraduate students. After professional experience in a number of countries, his current work includes nurses at all levels where he has the opportunity to teach and facilitate learning in a wide range of settings. By incorporating personal philosophies of care and caring into the facilitated sessions he can support reflection, promote awareness and stimulate the development of personal caring attitudes in relation to the individual practitioner's daily experiences.

Reflection and reflective practice have been central to Philip's research, which incorporated the principles of confluent education linked to the professional socialisation of nurses.

This 4th edition has been updated by Philip from the original work by Lioba Howatson-Jones.

Dr Lioba Howatson-Jones was Senior Lecturer in the School of Nursing at Canterbury Christ Church University, where she taught pre-registration, post-registration, Master's and PhD students. Lioba's clinical nursing background is mainly in acute and radiology nursing and practice development. Her research interests are in exploring nurses' learning and academic development. Lioba has published on these and clinical topics since 1999.

Introduction

This book provides suggestions for developing analytical skills through different ways of using personal and professional *reflection* for learning and developing as a practitioner. The purpose of the book is to introduce you, the novice or more experienced practitioner, to a number of models and frameworks for reflection, as well as ways of integrating personal and professional reflective insights to help support safe and effective practice. The aim is to assist you to develop a sense of agency in your own learning by broadening the scope and depth of your reflection to include biographical aspects. The reason for this is to help you to develop a life-wide (as well as a life-long) view of learning and reflection, which can sustain your practice and you as a practitioner.

This book should be viewed as offering practical guidance to becoming reflective. It will be particularly useful for those starting out on such a process or wanting to try different methods. As you and your reflection develop, so too will your interest and reading to include ever more complex concepts and professional experience. The following chapters will encourage you to examine your experience and learning within the reflective process – through case studies, scenarios and activities that are rooted in the realities of practice and learning. This will help you to cope with the uncertainty of developing as a professional in a constructive way.

Chapter 1 sets the scene, showing how reflection has come about and its relevance for the new student and developing practitioner. It identifies some potential benefits that reflection can bring for the person, profession, patients/clients, organisation and society. It is important for the novice and experienced practitioner to recognise the significance of reflection for effective practice and development of professional knowledge, particularly the fundamentals of practice.

Chapter 2 emphasises that learning not only takes place through formal courses or instruction, but also extends into all areas of life. This chapter invites you to review some of these areas reflectively in order to extend learning potential. The focus here is on the types of knowledge produced through this reflective process, and the ways of knowing that can develop, which are crucial to life-long learning.

Chapter 3 introduces you, the student or developing practitioner, to autobiographical reflection as a means of helping to advance nursing knowledge in more diverse ways. In this chapter you are invited to integrate autobiographical reflection and learning with a sense of your developing identity, as well as to reflect on aspects of life that may reveal societal issues.

Chapter 4 introduces some of the wide range of reflective models and frameworks that you, as the student or practitioner, can draw upon when first starting to structure and frame their reflections. The chapter also considers the strengths and limitations of these, to help you to choose appropriately.

Chapter 5 introduces you, as the student or developing practitioner, to concepts of reflection as a transitional space in which you are encouraged to explore, develop and grow. As you progress, more will be expected in terms of knowledge, skills and decision-making. How a transitional space can draw out reflection and learning is a particular focus here.

Chapter 6 examines how student nurses and developing practitioners can influence their experiences, and how those experiences might influence them. It focuses on the role of reflexivity in developing opportunities for learning.

Chapter 7 invites you to cultivate a reflective approach to daily experience, and integrate what you are learning. It is important for students to be able to acknowledge limitations within their knowledge as well as to own potential mistakes, and this chapter focuses on how to respond to fallibility – in yourself and in other professionals.

Chapter 8 considers how guided reflection, and reflecting with others, can deepen your understanding and analysis of situations, experiences and decisions, and offer support. The chapter also introduces ways of dealing with emotional residues of caring work.

Chapter 9 explores the purpose of reflective writing and introduces you, the student, to a variety of techniques. You are encouraged to try out some different exercises to help develop this skill. Some examples of reflective writing are discussed.

Chapter 10 looks at the possibilities new media offer for reflecting with others. It explores potential benefits and pitfalls, and identifies how to develop your own digital story on which to reflect.

Chapter 11 emphasises the intense nature of critical reflection and its relevance to developing the skill of criticality. You are encouraged to consider your personal contributions and those of others to the development and outcomes of experiences.

NMC's Standards of Proficiency for Registered Nurses

The Nursing and Midwifery Council (NMC) has standards of proficiency that have to be met by applicants to different parts of the nursing and midwifery register. These standards are what they deem as being necessary for the delivery of safe, effective nursing and midwifery practice.

This book includes the latest standards for 2018 onwards, taken from *Future Nurse: Standards of Proficiency for Registered Nurses* (NMC, 2018a).

Learning features

Learning by reading text is not always easy. Therefore, to provide variety and assist with the development of independent learning skills, and the application of theory to practice, this book contains activities, example stories, scenarios (some with questions), case studies, concept summaries, further reading and useful websites to enable you to participate in your own learning. You will need to develop your own study skills and 'learn how to learn' to get the best from the material. The book cannot provide all the answers, but rather provides a framework for your learning.

The activities in the book will help you in particular to make sense of, and learn about, the material being presented. Some activities ask you to reflect on aspects of practice, or your experience of it, or the people or situations you encounter. *Reflection* is an essential skill in nursing, and it helps you to understand the world around you and often to identify how things might be improved. Other activities will help you develop key graduate skills such as your ability to *think critically* about a topic in order to challenge received wisdom, or your ability to *research a topic* and *find appropriate information and evidence*, and to be able to make decisions using that evidence in situations that are often difficult and time pressured. Communication and working as part of a team are core to all nursing practice, and some activities will ask you to think about your *communication skills* to help develop these.

All the activities require you to take a break from reading the text, think through the issues presented and carry out some independent study, possibly using the internet. Where appropriate, there are sample answers presented at the end of each chapter, and these will help you to understand more fully your own reflections and independent study. You will gain most from the activities if you try to complete them yourself before reading the suggested answers. Remember, academic study will always require independent work; attending lectures will never be enough to be successful on your programme, and these activities will help to deepen your knowledge and understanding of the issues under scrutiny and give you practice at working on your own.

You might want to think about completing these activities as part of your personal development plan (PDP) or portfolio. After completing the activity, write it up in your PDP or portfolio in a section devoted to that particular skill, then look back over time to see how far you have developed. You can also do more of the activities for a key skill in which you have identified a weakness; this will help build your skill and confidence in this area.

There is a glossary of terms at the end of the book, which provides an interpretation of some of the terminology in the context of the subject of the book.

All chapters have further reading and useful websites listed at the end, with notes to show you why we think they will be helpful to you. The websites will also help you to remain up to date with developments in this aspect of practice, as awareness of key issues grows and policies develop.

We hope that you find this book helpful in developing your professional practice and that it challenges you to ensure that you provide care and support that reduces the risk of vulnerability, and promotes dignity, respect and a positive quality of life. Good luck with your studies!

Chapter 1

What is meant by reflection and reflective practice?

NMC Standards of Proficiency for Registered Nurses

This chapter will address the following platforms and proficiencies:

Platform 1: Being an accountable professional

1.3   Understand and apply the principles of courage, transparency and the professional duty of candour, recognising and reporting any situations, behaviours or errors that could result in poor care outcomes.

1.17   Take responsibility for continuous self-reflection, seeking and responding to support and feedback to develop their professional knowledge and skills.

Platform 6: Improving safety and quality of care

6.3   Comply with local and national frameworks, legislation and regulations for assessing, managing and reporting risks, ensuring the appropriate action is taken.

Chapter aims

After reading this chapter you will be able to:

- define reflection and reflective practice;
- understand the relevance of reflection in nursing;
- identify benefits for the person, profession, patients/clients, organisation and society;
- understand the requirements of the Nursing and Midwifery Council's Code (NMC, 2018b);
- understand the nature of accountability and reflection and how this relates to the 6 Cs of nursing;
- understand which legislation could impact on the nurse's role;
- begin to explore personal and professional forms of reflection.

Introduction

Scenario 1.1: Heather's reflection on professional practice

Heather was working on a learning disability nursing placement in the community in the second year of her mental health nurse preparation programme. She enjoyed the placement, although some aspects could be challenging such as when an independent living resident was emotionally distressed. Heather's practice supervisor Barbara was often busy, and Heather frequently took her concerns home.

Yesterday Heather and Barbara had visited 25-year-old Jack who has autism and had moved out of the family home to gain more independence. This was the first time that Barbara had met Jack because he had been under the care of Mo, another nurse, previously. Barbara checked that Jack was coping with the change to his circumstances and that he had food in the house. Jack made Barbara and Heather a cup of tea and they talked about his week. During the discussion Jack spoke about Mo, saying he liked him a lot. He said that Mo had met him on Friday night when Jack was out with friends at the pub. Jack bought the drinks with his allowance, something Jack said he did often when Mo met him. After some further talk about other aspects of Jack's week Barbara and Heather left.

On the way to the car Heather asked Barbara if it was acceptable for nurses to socialise with service users like Jack. Barbara said this was just Mo's way of helping Jack assimilate into society and the local community and told Heather not to worry about it. She explained where they were going next and got in the car.

When Heather got home that evening she could not stop thinking about her meeting with Jack and what Barbara had said. Heather tried to reflect on the situation but felt confused and unsure what to do. She was concerned that Mo had taken advantage of his position and behaved unprofessionally with Jack, allowing him to spend his allowance on Mo. Heather was also uneasy that Barbara did not appear concerned about this. Heather wondered whether this was because she was not yet fully aware of the policies and procedures used in the learning disability setting, or whether Barbara was covering for a colleague. Heather, therefore, felt she could not approach Barbara about her anxieties.

Heather, along with fellow mental health students, participated in an ongoing support group throughout the programme. She decided to discuss the issue with the group at the next session. The group was facilitated by Said who asked her some reflective questions about what she was thinking and feeling, the evidence for this, and the alternatives and potential consequences of following these. Heather concluded that following the process for raising concerns about practice was the course of action she would take, with the help of her personal tutor.

As illustrated in Scenario 1.1, although we need to believe that healthcare profession-als' intentions are honourable and that they do not mean to intentionally harm service users, reports, unfortunately, suggest otherwise and we should be alert and mindful of things that happen. A small study among psychologists responsible for supporting ser-vice users with learning disability by Hewitt (2014) suggests that 25% of clients referred to psychology services reported some form of abuse, with 13% of the perpetrators being staff, the most prevalent abuse being psychological, sexual and physical.

Professionals are sometimes fallible and the example above is offered as an illustra-tion of the importance of reflection in helping to make sense of things and make effective decisions. The disturbing findings of the independent inquiry into the Mid Staffordshire NHS Foundation Trust failings (Francis, 2013) highlight some of the potential consequences of ignoring concerns about care (see Further reading at the end of the chapter). The report identified that patients' needs were ignored, that they were not treated with compassion and that when concerns were raised they were not acted upon. In response to this indictment of care standards, the Chief Nurse for England, Jane Cummins, in association with the Department of Health (2012), devel-oped some principles for care and compassion described as the 6 Cs.

When reading the example above, a number of thoughts may go through your mind: 'Why did the practice supervisor find the contact between Mo and Jack acceptable?', 'Why did the student nurse not ask what the policy was about socialising?', 'Why did the practice supervisor not check what Heather's concerns were?' and 'What might have been done differently?' Even if reflection is not a familiar concept to you, par-ticularly when starting your nurse preparation programme, this kind of curiosity and questioning can form the basis of personal reflection. So, this chapter begins by setting the scene of what reflection is and its relevance for the new student as well as the more experienced practitioner. It contextualises reflection and **reflective practice** through tracing some of the main historical roots and key developments to help establish its importance in the nursing profession. Patient safety, accountability, empathy, errors and near misses are examples of practice issues that can be influenced by reflection (or a lack thereof). The chapter further emphasises the significance of reflection for effec-tive, professional practice and development of professional knowledge in accordance with legislation, the NMC's Code (2018b) and the 6 Cs. The chapter concludes by con-sidering accountability issues and the relationship to professional and personal forms of reflection. You are invited throughout the chapter to complete a variety of activities and consider several case studies and scenarios. This will help you to start reflecting if you are a novice, or to develop reflection if you are a more experienced practitioner.

What is reflection?

In the past decades, reflection has been defined in various ways: as accessing previous experience that helps to develop 'tacit knowledge' and 'intuitive knowledge' (Johns and Freshwater, 2005); a continuous cycle in which experience and reflection on experiences are interrelated (Chong, 2009); a transformative process that changes individuals and their actions (Ghaye and Lillyman, 2010); a way to reach awareness of how and why things have occurred (Johns, 2013), and that reflection should be critical in nature and focus on consistency and inconsistency of actual care delivery with values, standards and regulations (de Vries and Timmins, 2016).

Although the formal definitions of reflection may seem quite abstract and academic, we should remember that reflection is not unusual. We do it in the car, on the train, cooking a meal, while undertaking exercise, in the bath, and during and after conversations, basically wherever we can find mental and physical space to take a moment to think about things. Take a little time out now to think about what you did today and complete Activity 1.1.

Activity 1.1   Reflection

Spend a little time reviewing what you have done today. As a tip, you could think about the day as a whole, jot down things that come to mind and then prioritise them so that you can answer the following questions:

- What particular aspects were significant and why?
- When and where did you find yourself thinking about something in more depth?
- Can you track changes to your thinking?
- What do you think about the issue now?

There is an outline answer to this activity at the end of the chapter.

When completing the activity, you may have identified another way that you would have liked to have done things, or other things you might have liked to have said (or left unsaid), or you may have arrived at a different conclusion. However, as a professional, this 'reflection' or 'thinking things over' will probably need to become more focused and structured in order to learn from the things we experience. Two important frameworks, the NMC's Code (2018b) and the 6 Cs, should inform the professional nurse's reflection and could be used to structure the reflective process (please refer to Chapter 4 for more information on reflective models).

Literature refers to 'tacit knowledge' as having a common understanding about something, whereas 'intuitive knowledge' means being sensitive to links with previous experience. In the example at the start of the chapter Heather is trying to make sense of things through reflecting on her own and with others to identify possible explanations for Mo's behaviour and the effects on Jack. Reflection is a way of examining your experience, explanations and alternative approaches to doing things. It may happen as part of an activity or later, when you have more time to think about what you have experienced. What is required is an open and enquiring mind that can accept the possibility of several different explanations. Reflection means that thoughts of significant aspects of an experience are reconsidered and other explanations are contemplated. For the more experienced practitioner, reflection may reach greater depths because there is more knowledge and a wider range of experience to examine. For example, reflection may be triggered by a different response to a routine action and proceed beyond the immediate situation to consider knowledge, personal values and personal practice as well as the values and practice of others. When considering Heather's situation in Scenario 1.1, you might want to start the reflective process by considering the NMC's Code (2018b). For Scenario 1.1, two sections of the Code are particularly relevant: *Preserve safety* and *Promote professionalism and trust.* Please take some time to read the Code and you will find that the first section addresses raising concerns and the second focuses on professional behaviour. Also relevant for this scenario is to think about what legislation would be appropriate, for example you might want to consider issues of safeguarding as identified in the Care Act 2014, the Safeguarding Vulnerable Groups Act 2006, the Mental Capacity Act 2005 and the Care Standards Act 2000. You might also want to consider how the 6 Cs are articulated in everyday care and professional values. It may be worthwhile realising that, although the 6 Cs form the value base for the nursing and midwifery professional, application relies on personal interpretation.

The 6 Cs are defined as follows:

- Care

  Care is our core business and that of our organisations, and the care we deliver helps the individual person and improves the health of the whole community. Caring defines us and our work. People receiving care expect it to be right for them, consistently, throughout every stage of their life.

- Compassion

  Compassion is how care is given through relationships based on empathy, respect and dignity. It can also be described as intelligent kindness and is central to how people perceive their care.

- Competence

  Competence means all those in caring roles must have the ability to understand an individual's health and social needs, and the expertise, clinical and technical knowledge to deliver effective care and treatments based on research and evidence.

- Communication

  Communication is central to successful caring relationships and to effective team working. Listening is as important as what we say and do, and essential for 'no decision about me without me'. Communication is the key to a good workplace with benefits for those in our care and staff alike.

- Courage

  Courage enables us to do the right thing for the people we care for, to speak up when we have concerns, and to have the personal strength and vision to innovate and to embrace new ways of working.

- Commitment

  A commitment to our patients and populations is a cornerstone of what we do. We need to build on our commitment to improve the care and experience of our patients, to take action to make this vision and strategy a reality for all and meet the health, care and support challenges ahead.

  (DH and NHS Commissioning Board, 2012: 13)

You may want to think about the need for Heather to have courage in taking this further. Why would this need courage? If you were in Heather's position, would you also find it courageous to address the situation? Why would this be? You might also have considered that Heather started reflecting when going home from the situation and that sharing her concerns in the support group, and reflecting on them in more detail, consolidated her decision-making about what were the best options for Jack, for the organisation and for her. What would your thoughts have been if you had been in Heather's situation? Would you have raised this situation in the support group? Why? Try to explicitly identify what you think the problem is? In your opinion, how do you think the situation should or could be resolved? Please attempt Activity 1.2, remembering to write down your reflections as you work through it.

Activity 1.2   Critical thinking

Read the example at the start of the chapter again and consider how/why reflection is relevant here. Please write these points down. Now consider which legislation must be considered, and which elements of the NMC's Code (2018b) and which of the 6 Cs are relevant to the case. Once you've thought about and identified the elements that are appropriate to the example, try to take the activity a step further by writing down why you think they are appropriate. Use the relevant documentation to support your ideas.

There is an outline answer at the end of the chapter.

Having worked through Activity 1.2, you might think differently about Scenario 1.1. You might have found the ramifications of the situation somewhat overwhelming, but bear in mind that this is the perfect opportunity to explore your personal values in relation to your professional and legal responsibilities. In working through these scenarios, sometimes other explanations might need to be imagined – particularly for the inexperienced practitioner – and confirmed with someone more experienced. It is important to separate fantasy (what you might like to happen) from the reality of what is possible or likely, for example, imagining the potential reaction of a client or patient, or considering possible consequences of a particular act. Please look at Scenario 1.2 and see if you can gain further understanding of the role of imagination in reflection. You are asked to identify some of these features after reading Scenario 1.2.

Scenario 1.2: Bruce's experience of using imagination as a novice practitioner

Bruce was working on an endoscopy unit in the second year of his nurse preparation programme. The work was fast paced, requiring a large number of admissions and documentation to be completed quickly to get people ready. Today Bruce was working with his practice supervisor Naomi in the endoscopy theatre. They were assisting with a *colonoscopy* list. Biju, a 75-year-old man, was the first patient and was quite nervous. After checking the documentation to make sure that they had the right patient, the proper preparation had been completed and Biju had consented to the procedure, Naomi asked Bruce to help reassure Biju while she inserted a cannula into his left hand and started to administer the prescribed sedative and *analgesia*. Bruce spoke to Biju about his travels before starting university and a memorable visit to India. Biju drifted off and the procedure started.

The consultant Robert called Bruce across to look through the colonoscope at various stages, explaining the anatomy that Bruce was observing. Towards the end of the procedure Robert again called Bruce to take a look because he had found a lesion. Bruce observed Robert taking a number of images of what he had found. Robert told Bruce that he thought this was a bowel cancer and that he would need to tell Biju when he had recovered after the procedure.

Bruce imagined that Biju would be upset and worried when given this news. Bruce had previously worked on a surgical ward and knew that bowel cancer patients often had to have a *colostomy* formed and Bruce imagined that Biju would find this difficult to accept. As Bruce had helped Biju relax at the beginning of the procedure, Naomi suggested it would help Biju to see a familiar face afterwards, so asked Bruce to complete his aftercare. This would also allow Bruce to be present at and observe the breaking of bad news.

Robert came to speak to Biju at the end of the morning. By this time Biju's daughter Bindu had arrived. Bruce stayed to observe Robert telling Biju the bad news of suspected bowel cancer and what further processes would follow. He expected Biju and his daughter to get upset, but they remained remarkably calm. After Robert had gone, Bruce told Biju and Bindu how sorry he was about the result. He was surprised

(Continued)

> (Continued)
>
> when they both smiled at him and said this was 'karma'. Biju stated he had had a good life and this would help him in the next one.
>
> Bruce reflected on this on his way home. He decided he needed to gather more information about different religions and cultures to aid his understanding because Biju's reaction was so different to what he had expected. This information would help his learning about breaking bad news to different people.

Following Scenario 1.2, Activity 1.3 asks you to reflect on Bruce's experience with Biju.

Activity 1.3   Reflection

- What are the significant features in Scenario 1.2 and why?
- If you were an experienced nurse, how might your reflective imagination have differed from Bruce's?

There are outline answers to these questions at the end of the chapter.

Having read Scenario 1.2 and answered the questions at the end, you will be able to see that reflection using imagination can identify several different strands of a situation, and how this might be relevant to practice. We return to the role of imagination in reflection in Chapter 3. Scenario 1.2 also illustrates the importance of reflecting on events.

The chapter now proceeds to define what reflective practice is.

What is reflective practice?

In addition to the different definitions of reflection indicated at the start of this chapter, Rolfe (2011) suggests that reflective practice is a process that develops understanding of what it means to be a practitioner, and Jasper (2003) suggests that it links theory and practice through the practitioner consciously thinking through the experience. This is an important activity for novice practitioners to help develop an understanding of their role and support the learning of new skills. To do so, reflection can occur within the experience or by looking back at the experience. Schön (1991) identifies these as reflection-in-action and reflection-on-action. Thinking about things requires knowledge of theory to develop answers, but theory needs to be mapped on to a situation in order to use it for problem solving. Reflection-in-action refers to knowing what to do and making a difference within a given situation – in Heather's example, she identified a situation 'in the moment' and attempted to address it, but, due to lack of knowledge or confidence, was not able to follow it through. Reflection-on-action, however, means examining some of those 'in the moment' decisions for the possibility of other choices and ways of acting, and how these insights might shape and develop future practice. This happens after the situation, just as Heather had thought about the situation of Jack and Mo in the evening once she was home. Besides questioning the actual Jack/Mo situation, Heather could have thought about why she was not able to press the discussion with Barbara, and what she could have done differently to address her questions or misgivings more satisfactorily in the future. Reflection often contains multiple levels of exploration; as seen from Heather's example she reflected on the actual situation and whether the contact between Jack and Mo was professional. However, at a more personal level she could reflect on how she had discussed her reservations with Barbara and how she could have done this differently. This is where the Courage C and the Communication C could be explained. Did Heather feel intimidated through her lack of knowledge about policy? Perhaps she felt uncomfortable raising questions of professional practice about a colleague with whom she had regularly worked? These elements of reflection are more personal and lead to professional growth and are discussed in later chapters.

At this point we move away from reflection-in-action and reflection-on-action to focus more on problem solving, which can take the form of rational thinking based on protocols and procedures. However, simply imitating role-modelled behaviour in dealing with situations is a form of non-reflective learning (Jarvis, 2006). For example, when undertaking a drug round, if the practitioner is mainly intent on fulfilling the requirements of the five rights of drug administration, through checking the right dose, right drug, right patient, right time and right route, and does not reflectively consider their actions, knowledge or the patient, this does not develop learning. What aids learning is looking beyond the basic actions to examine understanding and personal responses. Reflective practice requires careful consideration of knowledge and ideas.

As illustrated above, reflective practice considers practice as a 'whole' which consists of different layers and elements that cannot always be rationalised. Individuals are unique, and human factors may be uncertain, even messy. Reflective practice is, therefore, based on experience and intuitive learning of which you may not be aware until you need to respond to a situation. Although it may seem easier for some practitioners to respond to situations because they have greater experience to draw on, reflection always takes courage and commitment. Capturing such learning by bringing it into awareness through reflecting on practice is an important part of developing understanding, skill and competence as a practitioner at any stage of your career. This is especially true when the ideal does not match the reality of the situation – what Argyris and Schön (1978) call espoused theories versus theories in use. Espoused theories form the basis of protocols and procedures that indicate how practice should proceed. Theories in use can be subconscious customs and practices or professional knowing from reflective practice, and are therefore considered to be 'in action'. An example of a discrepancy between espoused theory and theories in use would be having learned an evidence-based hand-washing technique, such as the Ayliffe technique, and successfully passing on the related assessments, but then taking shortcuts in the busyness of a shift, such as using the full Ayliffe technique only after what you consider to be 'dirty' procedures. This practice, although incorrect, might be wrongly perceived as 'acceptable'. Novice practitioners sometimes identify differences between 'theory' and 'practice' or even differences between practice supervisors. By using critical reflection, we can become aware of such discrepancies in our own actions, re-evaluate the quality of our work and develop alternative behaviour. This is where the courage and commitment, as mentioned earlier, come into play; critical reflection can be an uncomfortable process, in which individuals become aware of and confront previously unconscious qualities, behaviour or tendencies in themselves that can be distressing. In this way reflective practice can contribute to organisational learning through its members.

The idea of critical reflection can be taken a step further. Knowledge derived from practice does not add to professional knowledge unless it has been reflected on for its significance (Eraut, 2001). For example, as a novice practitioner you may have worked with healthcare assistants and your practice supervisor. You may have observed and been involved in completing a care element, such as a bed bath, with both at some point. You may even have been aware of some differences between them in how the care was completed. However, unless you reflect on this and reach some conclusions about the significance of the differences, the care will remain a task that was completed in different ways, and perhaps not the expression of nursing knowledge and values that it might have been. The learning and articulation of values embedded within this will be lost. Equally, an experienced practitioner who may have to complete similar tasks can gain greater insight and knowledge through reflecting on how the tasks themselves might be the same and yet different each time they are performed, and what knowledge and values are being used and maybe even generated, in order to avoid simple repetition of experience that does not constitute learning.

Now apply some of the principles of reflective practice to your own practice by completing Activity 1.4.

Activity 1.4   Critical thinking

When you are next in practice and in a nursing situation, try to consider the following:

- What is going on?
- What knowledge are you using?
- What values are you drawing upon and articulating in the situation?

- What decisions are you making?
- How have you come to those decisions?
- Are you trying out different things?
- What is changing your thinking, if anything?
- How are the above relevant to the 6 Cs?

Allow an interval of at least a day between the situation and reflecting on it further. Now ask yourself the same questions again.

- Have your answers changed and, if so, how?
- What learning are you taking forward from this?

It is useful to keep asking yourself these questions and to maintain a reflective diary to track your learning and development.

It might help to document this activity by using the pro forma offered at the end of the chapter.

As this activity is based on your own experiences, there is no outline answer at the end of the chapter.

Chapter 7 picks up the theme of reflective practice again by looking at what constitutes the reflective practitioner. Having defined what reflection and reflective practice are, this chapter now proceeds to take a brief look at the development of reflection and its relevance in the context of nursing.

History and development of reflection in the context of nursing

It might be surmised that early pioneers of nursing (such as Florence Nightingale) potentially came to different conclusions of what was needed in terms of sanitation in hospitals, through possibly reflecting on the problem; this is illustrated in the preface to *Notes on Nursing: What it is and what it is not* (Nightingale, 1969). Nightingale states *Every day sanitary knowledge, or the knowledge of nursing, or in other words, of how to put the constitution in such a state that it will have no disease, or that it can recover from disease, takes a higher place* (Nightingale, 1969). One could argue that Nightingale's interpretation of sanitary fits with Jasper's (2003) concept of reflection linking theory and practice through conscious thought and Rolfe's (2011) idea that reflective practice is a process that develops understanding of what it means to be a practitioner. What is clear is that the possibilities for reflection begin to appear in nursing through research studies that explore different types of nursing knowledge.

For example, Carper (1978) identified patterns of knowing that looked further than a medical model of disease management to where nurses discovered new nursing theories through working out their ideas. Benner's (1984) influential work started to explain how nurses developed their knowledge in practice, and Watson (1988, 2008) recognised the importance of previous practice in shaping nurses' perceptions of knowledge and urged that nurses also needed to develop new insights. Schön (1991) suggested reflection as getting to the heart of how professionals think in action.

Changes in nurses' basic preparation have meant that there has been an increasing focus on reflection as a tool for teaching and learning. Since the early 1990s, interest in reflection as a concept, and its contribution within nurse education, have grown (Pierson, 1998). In 1994, the United Kingdom Central Council (UKCC), nursing's regulatory body at the time, pronounced that all nurses needed to maintain a portfolio of evidence of learning activity and listed reflection as an essential component of this activity (UKCC, 1994). This requirement has been updated by the Nursing and Midwifery Council (NMC, 2017), which makes it clear that reflection on the outcome of any type of learning is essential for maintaining knowledge, skills and competence as a nurse, and has been incorporated into the NMC's revalidation process. More recently, debates about the future shape of caring suggest that what is essential in the preparation and education of nurses is developing good decision-making skills (Willis, 2015). Reflection can help with this by examining the evidence and alternative courses of action and thereby coming to an informed decision. Thus reflection, in the context of nursing, is now a foundation for learning that takes place both inside and outside the classroom.

The discourse between the novice and experienced practitioner is part of an ongoing reflective dialogue that continues to take nursing practice forward through the new insights that are revealed within such discussions (Johns, 2012). Thus, the student nurse and the experienced practice supervisor can contribute to nursing knowledge in dynamic ways through interaction. For example, questioning and exploring what is known about a situation or topic, brings what is unknown also into view and both can be considered as part of developing a wider understanding as well as critically considering what values are brought to bear on a situation and why. This is an important part of developing the profession, as you can see from this case study illustrating some dialogue between a student and a practice supervisor.

Case study: Student and practice supervisor dialogue

Student: *I have never come across anyone with a learning disability. How do I talk to them?*

Practice supervisor: *How do you like to be talked to?*

Student:	*I like people to use my first name and for us to share our views on the topic of conversation.*
Practice supervisor:	*That is a good way to talk to someone. Ask them to tell you a bit about themselves and share their views. What have you learned about communication in your preparation programme?*
Student:	*We have learned about how to build therapeutic relationships using verbal and non-verbal communication and about empathy and using the 6 Cs. But I am not sure how they might respond.*
Practice supervisor:	*We don't know how anyone might respond – we have to take our cues from them. What is your main concern?*
Student:	*That I might upset them and not know what to do.*
Practice supervisor:	*One way of avoiding this is to learn to read emotional cues or what is sometimes called 'emotional intelligence'. If you attune yourself to others' emotional cues you can start to work out how they are feeling and responding to what you are saying. When I started nursing I found it hard to talk to people because I was very shy. I still am shy, but what has helped me is learning to move beyond my own feelings by becoming aware of others' emotional feelings and responding accordingly. This is part of emotional intelligence.*
Student:	*I think we had a lecture about emotional intelligence and watched a video about empathy.*
Practice supervisor:	*Start talking to one of our residents today by finding out a bit about each other. You could start by saying what your interests are and ask them about theirs. Then revisit your notes from that lecture and reflect on what you have learned today. We will discuss your reflection about this tomorrow.*

The case study of student and practice supervisor dialogue illustrates how thinking about and reflecting on practice issues is an important way for professional knowledge to develop. 'Socratic questioning', which asks for thinking, is an essential part of this learning process. The idea of developing understanding and knowledge of nursing through reflection brings benefits for the nurse and patient. Some of these benefits are explored in the next section of the chapter, which looks at the benefits of reflection.

Benefits of reflection

Reflection can help us to affirm some actions but can also trigger us to consider correcting other actions. In doing so it may enable us to translate successful strategies into new situations, and thus continue to develop them. Equally, when reflection reveals problems with an action taken, it will enable you to avoid using that action in similar circumstances again or allow you to consider other corrections. It can help you to identify the causes of errors or potential errors, called near misses, thereby promoting patient safety and learning as recommended in the Francis (2013) report. From such a perspective, reflection can help to raise your confidence in your developing abilities and highlight things to avoid. Some benefits from reflection for the individual practitioner, the organisation and the patient are summarised in Figure 1.1.

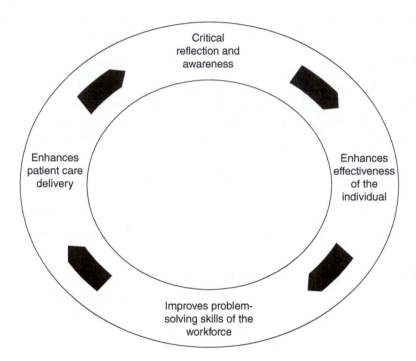

Figure 1.1 Benefits from reflection for the individual practitioner, the organisation and the patient

Reflection means making the familiar unfamiliar or looking at it with fresh eyes (Abrandt Dahlgren et al., 2004). You will be able to chart the development of your effectiveness in problem solving and delivery of patient care by using reflection throughout your nursing programme. Equally, as an experienced practitioner, reflection will help you to re-evaluate your personal effectiveness in problem solving and the management of patient care. Through the improving skills of the individual, the organisation benefits, as do the clients and patients for whom the organisation offers a service. Thus, reflection as practised by you would reflect across the profession throughout your lifetime as a nurse. By completing Activity 1.5, you will be able to consider in more detail some of the benefits reflection might have for you.

Activity 1.5   Reflection

As a student nurse you will need to learn clinical skills. Think about the first skill you learned.

- What were the highlights of learning this skill?
- What were the problems?
- How did you deal with any existing or potential problems?
- How did you feel about learning the skill at the time?
- How did you feel about putting it into practice with a real person for the first time?
- Did your practice change in the live setting and, if so, why?
- What do you think about your practice of the skill now, after reflecting on it through these questions?
- What learning are you taking forward from this?

If you are an experienced practitioner consider the same questions in relation to decision-making and management skills.

There is an outline answer to this activity at the end of the chapter.

Having identified your learning of the skill through Activity 1.5 and your evaluation of it, you will now get a clearer picture of your knowledge and ability. These are important aspects of your personal responsibility and accountability. We now move on to consider how accountability relates to reflection.

Accountability and reflection

The professional code of conduct for nurses and midwives expects nurses to maintain their knowledge in order to provide safe and effective practice (NMC, 2018b). Working within the boundaries of the code is a part of the standard of professional behaviour expected of nurses and nursing practice. As suggested earlier, simply receiving new ideas does not translate into becoming knowledgeable. Reflection is needed to take new concepts and understand how to use them. Therefore, if as a nurse you are expected to maintain your knowledge, it follows that thinking and reflecting on that knowledge and what you do are part of your accountability as a nurse. Scenarios 1.3 and 1.4 look at Mandy's responsibility and Sarah's accountability as a way of illustrating the process of reflecting on these aspects within learning from practice. After reading Scenario 1.3, in Activity 1.6 you are asked to identify what aspects you might need to reflect on and what your response might be.

Scenario 1.3: Mandy's responsibility

Mandy was in the second year of her nursing programme. She had been working in a day surgery unit that encompassed a pre-assessment area, ward and theatre suite, with the ward phone as the central contact point. The unit was busy with people coming and going, and the phone ringing with relatives enquiring about whether patients were ready to come home, or doctors asking for information. In one such phone call, a doctor asked Mandy to pass a message to the theatre staff about a certain instrument that should be available for the afternoon theatre list. Unfortunately, Mandy was distracted by a patient who started vomiting and needed her assistance, and she forgot to pass the message on.

When the afternoon began, a very angry nurse rang from the theatre suite to ask why the message about the specialised instrument had not been passed on. The patient's procedure had to be cancelled because the necessary instrument could not be prepared in time.

The doctor came to apologise to the patient who was not very happy. The theatre staff were upset that they appeared inefficient. The ward manager wanted to know who had taken the message and not passed it on. Mandy was also upset when she realised it was her and thought what to do next.

Activity 1.6   Reflection

- If you were Mandy, what would you think about, what would you reflect on and what would be your response?
- How does Scenario 1.3 relate to the 6 Cs?

There are outline answers to these questions at the end of the chapter.

Now consider another day in Mandy's placement, again on the same unit. After reading Scenario 1.4 and Activity 1.7, you are asked to identify what aspects you might need to reflect on and what your learning might be.

Scenario 1.4: Whose accountability?

Mandy was working another shift on day surgery with her practice supervisor, Sarah. It was a Friday and the patients who had recovered from their procedures were eager to go home. Mandy was preparing one woman, who had undergone a *haemorrhoidectomy*, to go home. Haemorrhoidectomy can be quite a painful procedure and she was being sent home with some prescribed analgesia. The form of this analgesia was contraindicated in people who had asthma because it could induce an asthmatic episode. As Mandy was checking the medication and talking to the patient, she realised that the woman did have a history of asthma, although she did not take regular medication for it, only rarely needing to use an inhaler. Nevertheless, Mandy brought this to the attention of her practice supervisor, explaining that the drug had been prescribed and what she had found out about its contraindications. She reflected on what might have happened if she had not noticed. Would she have been responsible, as in the previous episode? Who would be accountable if the woman did subsequently suffer an asthmatic attack at home?

Activity 1.7   Reflection

- If you were Mandy, what would you reflect on in this situation?
- If you were Sarah, what would you reflect on in this situation? (If you are a novice practitioner, leave this part of the question.)
- How are responsibility and accountability assigned in Scenario 1.4?
- What might Mandy have learned from this situation?
- What might Sarah have learned from this situation? (If you are a novice practitioner, leave this part of the question.)

There are outline answers to these questions at the end of the chapter.

Scenarios 1.3 and 1.4 may have helped to give you a clearer idea of some of the differences between responsibility and accountability, and the role of reflection in helping to make sense of this. However, it is important to be mindful that responsibility and accountability go hand in hand and, although the two are separated in the examples above, we are accountable for taking responsibility for our actions. This is especially important when undertaking your nursing programme, because it can sometimes appear less clear in practice. Equally, as an experienced practitioner, reflecting on near-miss situations is important for adjusting practice. The chapter now proceeds to look at some personal and professional forms of reflection that can help with this.

Personal and professional forms of reflection

Journal writing is one method that has been used to develop reflective learning (Chirema, 2007). The private log, or blog, has become increasingly popular as a way of working out what has personally been learned. This is usually kept private and enters the public domain only when shared with a tutor through a progress review, or to inform assignment content when on a nurse preparation programme, as it forms part of the portfolio of evidence of learning. As technology has developed, the student on a nurse preparation programme may be asked to enter reflections on learning into an online *e-portfolio*, for example, PebblePad, with different templates such as structured reflection, a blog and curriculum vitae (CV) assigned to different aspects of the programme. The tutor has access to view the information only when this is shared by the student. The issue of using digital media for reflection is explored in more detail in Chapter 10. During your preparation programme you will perhaps have been asked to reflect on a variety of situations and scenarios, in the same way as you are in this book. You may also be asked to reflect on your assignments in the form of case studies, where you might include a review of your actions and contribution to the patient's care. Complete Activity 1.8 as a way of starting to think about recording your reflective learning. The issue of reflective writing is explored in more detail in Chapter 9.

Activity 1.8   Documenting reflection

Think about the main elements of your nursing programme. Write a reflection on your progress in each of these areas.

If you are an experienced practitioner, think about the main elements of your career development and write a reflection on your progress.

There is an outline answer to this activity at the end of the chapter.

For the experienced practitioner reflection involves thinking about the nursing identity and reconstructing experience in order to identify how to progress (Lindsay, 2006). As a novice to the nursing profession, you develop your own professional identity through undertaking the same process and this type of reflection examines aspects such as: *self-respect, hope, control, vulnerability, acceptance, loss* and *persistence* (Daley, 2001: 53).

For example, nursing someone who is dying may call into question our own mortality. Reconstructing the experience by looking at how we deal with loss might offer a way of examining how loss is interpreted in the context of dying and others' experience. This may stimulate reflective thinking about possible courses of action for helping others to face loss. Reflective writing may be entered into a private diary and considered privately during such 'working out'. Professional forms of reflection may take place individually or in a group through a variety of ways, such as clinical supervision or action learning. Different forms of reflecting with others are explored in greater detail in Chapter 8.

Chapter summary

This chapter has begun to define what reflection and reflective practice are and some of the contemporary drivers as to why reflection is so important for nursing practice. By offering activities that ask the novice and developing nurse to review thinking and practice, the chapter provides an opportunity for starting to develop reflection in relation to safe and effective nursing practice and decision-making. Through the inclusion of examples that help to illustrate the benefits of reflection, and the relationship between accountability and reflection, you are encouraged to start thinking about how this might be relevant to your learning and practice, as well as to working within a regulatory code. Different forms of reflection and reflective practice are explained further in later chapters.

Activities and Scenarios: Brief outline answers

Activity 1.1 Reflection (page 8)

Your answer might have considered:

- getting up;
- interaction with others at home;
- travelling to work;
- priorities for work;
- completing work;
- coming home.

When thinking about which aspects were significant and why, you might have first been alerted by triggered emotions, for example, anxiety, satisfaction or anger, which led you to consider the trigger; this might have been a decision that you had made or were finding difficult to make. From here you can then re-evaluate the situation.

Activity 1.2 Critical thinking (page 10)

In the example you could have decided that Heather is using courage, commitment and communication within the case to ensure that Jack's interests are safeguarded. The role of reflection has been to make sense of her feelings and then to look objectively at the options available to her using proper processes to ensure effectiveness. The fact that she is feeling uncomfortable about the situation with Jack and Mo should be a cue to explore the situation more fully. Jack is clearly a vulnerable adult and one of Heather's considerations would be to explore what legislation says about safeguarding, so you might want to look the Care Act 2014, the Safeguarding Vulnerable Groups Act 2006, the Mental Capacity Act 2005 and the Care Standards Act 2000. The Acts are unanimous in terms of the carer's responsibility in protecting the service user's interests. The 2012 National Institute for Health and Care Excellence (NICE) guideline, *Autism: The Nice Guideline on Recognition, Referral, Diagnosis and Management of Adults on the Autism Spectrum*, recommends that healthcare professionals should provide activities that promote social integration and minimise social isolation. One could, therefore, argue that Mo's intentions of going with Jack to the pub would be addressing this NICE recommendation. However, Mo's activity with Jack would not be considered professional conduct. From the perspective of the NMC's Code (2018b) sections concerning promoting professionalism (specifically items 20.1, 20.5, 20.6, 20.8 and 21.1), taking advantage of a service user, adhering to professional boundaries and accepting gifts, are considered to be a serious breach of professional conduct. Witnessing this places Heather in a position where she is obliged to escalate her concerns according to the NMC's Code sections about preserving safety (specifically items 16.1, 16.3, 7.1, 17.2 and 17.3). As Barbara did not seem particularly concerned about Mo's behaviour, when Heather talked to her, the responsibility is still with Heather to consider her next steps. As a student, Heather would have access to an escalating concerns policy and would be strongly advised to discuss the situation with her personal tutor or the liaison lecturer for the practice area.

Activity 1.3 Reflection on Scenario 1.2: Bruce's experience of using imagination as a novice practitioner (page 12)

The significant features in Scenario 1.2 that Bruce is likely to have reflected on are:

- the breaking of bad news;
- Biju's reaction;
- his knowledge of other religions and cultures.

Bruce used imagination to consider aspects where he did not have knowledge, namely:

- patient reaction to bad news;
- how he would respond if Biju asked him what the result of the procedure was;
- what happens next;
- the consequences of his lack of knowledge about other religions and cultures.

Which features would you reflect on if you were in Bruce's position?

As an experienced nurse your reflective imagination might have differed from Bruce's by identifying the significant features as:

- your accountability in this situation;
- how to offer additional support without causing offence.

You might have used imagination to consider the aspects you did not have knowledge of, such as:

- how the family might react to change;
- whether you have sufficient knowledge of other cultures and religions to understand Biju's response.

Although this activity is, fundamentally, about developing awareness of your own strengths and limitations, there are several items from the NMC's Code (2018b) that underpin this activity. It is worth considering these, for example, Section 2 *Prioritise people* (items 2.1, 2.2, 2.3, 2.4 and 2.6), which accentuates the need for partnership working and the role of the professional to empower the service user to take responsibility for their own health and well-being, and 20.7 of Section 20 which calls for the professional not to express their personal beliefs.

Activity 1.5 Reflection (page 19)

You might have thought about nursing skills such as taking a pulse and blood pressure: the difficulty of hearing the blood pressure when taking a manual measurement and of being nervous when faced with a real patient. As your skill has developed you may have identified some more subtle nuances, such as a slight variation in where the brachial artery might be located in different patients. You might have learned that a manual measurement is sometimes more accurate than an electronic one when blood pressure is significantly abnormal.

As an experienced practitioner you might have thought about decision-making in relation to problem solving, planning and implementing care. As your skill has developed you may have identified that you can do this quickly while dealing with competing demands. You might have considered management skills such as allocating the skill mix of staff and liaising with the hierarchy of management. You might have learned the strengths and weaknesses of your interpersonal skills and management strategies.

Activity 1.6 Reflection on Scenario 1.3: Mandy's responsibility (page 20)

In this scenario Mandy might think about talking to the doctor and theatre staff herself to take responsibility for the omission. She is likely to reflect on the circumstances that led her to forget and what she might have done differently, and how to avoid the omission in the future. Her initial response was to get upset when confronted by the ward manager, but thereafter she might have regained her confidence from having thought things through and reflecting on how to do things differently. The principle from the 6 Cs most affected is communication.

Activity 1.7 Reflection on Scenario 1.4: Whose accountability? (page 21)

In this scenario Mandy might reflect on what led her to identify the near miss. Sarah might reflect on the assessment of the patient, interprofessional communication, pharmacological knowledge and patient collaboration in care planning. In this scenario Mandy was responsible for completing the delegated task of preparing the patient for discharge and for reporting new information and any concerns. Sarah was accountable for acting on that information and for overseeing the care Mandy gave to the patient, including any drugs to take home. Mandy is likely to have learned that she has good assessment and observation skills which helped her to check information appropriately. Sarah might have learned that, no matter how experienced, professionals are fallible. She may also have learned that students can help to interrogate practice. When reflecting on Mandy's situation, it would be advisable to consider how this relates to the NMC's Code (2018b), for example, the section *Practise effectively* (items 8.1, 8.2, 8.3, 8.4, 8.5 and 8.6), which relates to sharing information and appropriate communication between team members.

Activity 1.8 Documenting reflection (page 22)

You might have written reflections on:

- developing graduate skills;
- knowledge and proficiency with information technology;
- developing essential clinical skills;
- practice;
- personal development planning.

As an experienced practitioner you might have written reflections on:

- developing leadership and management skills;
- developing your knowledge and proficiency in different practice situations;
- dealing with conflict and change.

To help document some of the reflection that you might have undertaken in completing the activities in this chapter, you might want to consider:

- description of experience;
- evaluation;
- analysis;
- future action.

The following pro forma is offered to help you begin to document reflection.

PRO FORMA FOR DOCUMENTING REFLECTION
Self-assessing experience:
Main points identified from reflection on the experience:
Learning points:
How will this learning be applied in the future?
Professional development achieved?

Further reading

Delves-Yates, C (2015) *Essential Clinical Skills for Nurses: Step by step.* London: Sage.

This book offers a step-by-step approach to developing clinical skills in any field.

Francis, R (2013) *Report of the Mid Staffordshire NHS Foundation Trust Public Inquiry: Executive summary.* London: HMSO. Retrieved from: www.midstaffspublicinquiry.com/sites/default/files/report/Executive%20summary.pdf

This report identifies the full scale of the deficits and failings in care and offers some recommendations for how these might be avoided in the future. You might like to relate your reading to your own practice and reflect on what further action to take.

Useful websites

www.supervisionandcoaching.com

This website offers a number of useful resources to help the reader to reflect. These can be found on the left-hand side. You are invited to try out the 'How reflective are you?' self-assessment.

www.autism.org.uk/about/adult-life/advocacy/mental-capacity-act-2005.aspx#

This 2007 *A Guide to the Mental Capacity Act* by the National Autistic Society provides an interpretation of the Mental Capacity Act 2005 in dealing with service users.

Chapter 2 Life-wide, life-long and life-deep learning and reflection

Chapter aims

By the end of this chapter you will be able to:

- define what is meant by life-wide, life-long and life-deep learning;
- identify the breadth of knowledge that a nurse needs to ensure is current;
- identify some of the contexts in which learning takes place;
- identify features of learning in formal and less formal ways;
- consider types of knowledge and ways of knowing;
- understand how the person learns through reflection.

Introduction

Scenario 2.1: Jenny's experience of sharing knowledge

....

Jenny had finished her first placement in her second year of the nursing programme and was back in the university studying her next module. The module was about acute care. During the module the tutor explained the need for vigilant assessment and the students were asked to investigate a variety of techniques and tools to undertake the assessment which encompassed a number of body systems. The scenarios offered were of mainstream surgical, medical and emergency situations which allowed the class to apply some of these strategies and techniques.

Jenny's placement had been in radiology, where she had observed a number of procedures such as an *aortic stent insertion* and *uterine embolisation*. These were newer procedures, offering alternatives to more invasive and major interventions, such as surgical aortic aneurysm repair and hysterectomy. Jenny reflected on ways in which some of the assessment principles might be relevant to this different environment and different groups of patients. She noted that, although the procedures were less invasive, they still represented acute care in that the patient was sedated and vulnerable to sudden major haemorrhage. Jenny discussed these different scenarios with her group during the group work and identified how the assessment strategies might be applied.

When the group was asked to give feedback about their work to the rest of the class, Jenny offered these alternative scenarios to help illustrate problem solving and application in a different care setting that, nevertheless, dealt with acute episodes within care. The tutor invited Jenny to explain more about the procedures in order to help expand the knowledge of the whole class – and her own, because she was not as familiar with the procedures as Jenny had been.

When reflecting upon this after class, Jenny realised that, no matter how knowledgeable a person may be, learning does not stop with a qualification. Equally, by explaining her learning about the procedures to others, Jenny was also able to perceive some gaps in her own knowledge in terms of the assessment strategies and tools at her disposal.

Learning can be defined as multi-dimensional in terms of where and how it takes place. Also, looking at the outcome skills suggested at the start of this chapter, it will be clear that developing and maintaining knowledge is not limited to clinical settings and patient or service user issues. Knowledge also needs to be current in relation to developments in policy and guidelines, technology, and political and health economic landscapes. Yet, learning is also a very individual process and what is carried forward may, perhaps, be truly gauged only by the people themselves. What is grasped may not always be what is taught. In Scenario 2.1, what is grasped is the need to assert a knowledge base, even if this differs from the examples being taught. The quality of the response received may influence whether this learning is taken forward or inhibited. To take ownership of learning requires an understanding of where and how learning can take place.

This chapter emphasises that learning not only takes place through formal courses or instruction, but also extends into all areas of life, a theme that is taken forward in Chapter 3. This chapter begins by defining what is meant by life-wide, life-long and life-deep learning and offers an example of each. We explore the contexts in which nurses might learn and consider them in terms of their levels of formality and learners' autonomy to design aspects of their own learning. At this point, it is important to accentuate the importance of taking responsibility for your own learning process and, wherever possible, being proactive in creating a learning environment. The chapter identifies different types of knowledge, how nurses come to know and how this relates to reflection. It concludes by summarising the interrelationship of reflection, developing an evidence base and informal learning.

Throughout the chapter, you will be invited to complete a variety of activities and consider a number of case studies and scenarios to enable you to examine the different contexts of your learning and analyse the progression of your learning.

What is life-wide learning?

Life-wide learning is learning that is not only limited to the classroom but also extends into many other areas of life (West et al., 2007). Banks et al. (2007) take this idea further and suggest that life-wide learning is broad and includes how we learn to be resilient and cope with challenge and adversity. Experience from these real-life situations allows us to transfer the knowledge we accumulate from one situation to another. They teach us to identify areas where we lack knowledge but also how to access the help of someone we trust in order to resolve the issue. Initially this support may be from parents, family or teachers but, after entering the nursing profession, could extend to include personal tutors or practice supervisors in clinical placements, whereas registered staff may turn to more experienced colleagues or unit leaders. To clarify, the idea of life-wide learning includes informal discussion, interest activities and learning within the family (Field, 2006). For example, we often discuss our views with others and in the process might learn a different perspective on a problem from their response, or even some new knowledge that they have learned and share with us. Becoming involved in an activity, such as sport, may involve learning the rules of the game or new techniques. Equally, incidental learning may occur during a formal preparation programme: for example, these could be skills such as typing, word processing or managing your time, or this learning could be more abstract, for example, developing professional attitudes such as care and compassion as suggested by the 6 Cs. These skills and attitudes may not be taught formally but are aspects that you are likely to absorb as part of completing the nursing programme. In Scenario 2.1, Jenny has learned that it is acceptable for professionals to admit they do not know something and allow others to take the lead in providing the information. Perhaps equally important, Jenny could identify a potential moment of learning and then create a learning environment that was beneficial to her and, in doing this, created a learning environment for the group. As individuals we should be able to define the different aspects of our lives that contribute to our learning. Consider the following case study of Paul's difficult encounter as an example of informal learning taking place within his social peer group.

Case study: Paul's difficult encounter

Paul was in the third year of his nursing programme. He lived in a rented house with two friends who were also on the programme. Paul was working in accident and emergency. During his shift one day, he had looked after a 13-year-old girl who had been brought in after taking an overdose of paracetamol. After recording her observations, he had tried to get hold of her mother. When her mother did arrive, she started shouting at her daughter, saying she was sick of her constant attention seeking and that she was going to put her into care. The mother and daughter were shouting so much that Paul had to ask the mother to wait in the waiting room. She replied that she washed her hands of her daughter and left. Paul was shocked and upset by this episode and came home troubled by it.

In the evening he broached the subject with his housemates, talking about the case but leaving out the names. He told them how he could not understand the mother's reaction. Why would she want to put her child into care? He wondered whether the reason the daughter had taken the overdose was because she felt unloved by her mother. He had also been disquieted by the reaction of some of the qualified staff who appeared not to take the girl seriously.

During their discussion it became clear that Paul's housemates had some alternative views which stemmed from their different experiences. They suggested that there might be a few reasons for the mother's reaction. Stress and exhaustion were obvious ones, if she felt she simply could not cope any longer. Paul's friend Rob explained how he had had a friend at school who would self-harm because of the pressure his stepfather put on him. At first, he could not understand it, until his friend explained that it was a bit like opening a release valve. The other housemate, Alex, who was on the mental health nursing programme, suggested that the mother and daughter might have been projecting behaviour on to each other because of the pain they were both experiencing. What he was trying to explain was that people can be manipulative for several reasons, not least because of the pain they feel and their poor self-esteem. Paul was thoughtful after this discussion and considered that perhaps his initial view was too simplistic. Projection was not something he knew much about and he thought it might be useful to explore further. He decided to read up on it to develop his understanding.

Having read this case study, you might have also questioned the daughter's and mother's actions. In addition, you might have perceived how the informal discussion within his house group developed Paul's thinking. By completing Activity 2.1 you will be able to review your own life-wide learning.

Activity 2.1 Critical thinking

For this activity, you need to think and list things that you have learned since you started with the nursing programme. Some of these things will have been developed due to the formal, taught sessions or tutorials. However, this activity needs you to focus on things that you have learned outside the formal sessions. Having done this, develop a map of your learning that extended beyond classroom-based learning. Try to form clusters of similar areas of learning and categorise them. You might want to consider situations involving:

- social learning;
- self-designed learning;
- leisure pursuit learning;
- family learning;
- incidental learning.

There is some guidance about this activity at the end of the chapter.

The map of your learning is likely to have illustrated how extensive your learning might be when considered outside the confines of the classroom and how this learning impacts on your professional and personal life. Many students specifically identify learning in areas such as assertiveness and communication that have benefitted them as student nurses, but can also identify the impact this has in their personal lives. Examining your learning in this way helps to analyse its progression. We now proceed to consider the relationship to life-long learning.

What is life-long learning?

Banks et al. (2007) suggest that life-long learning extends from childhood into old age and includes how we manage interpersonal interactions and our beliefs, and how we deal with new experiences. As you can imagine, we are often not aware or conscious of this learning. Similarly, Jarvis (2010) also considers life-long learning as a process of learning that continues across our lives. In addition, life-long learning is a professional reality for nurses because healthcare and the technologies that support it are constantly evolving. It is for this reason that life-long learning in healthcare often takes the form of professional development that is inextricably linked to practice development (Mason-Whitehead and Mason, 2008). The Nursing and Midwifery Council's (NMC, 2018b) Code advocates that nurses continue to learn not only to maintain the currency of their knowledge, but also to have an enquiring attitude to their practice and performance, for example, the section *Practice effectively* (items 6.1 and 6.2) which is part of *Platform 1: Being an accountable professional* of the NMC's *Standards of Proficiency for Registered Nurses* (NMC, 2018a), as presented in Scenario 2.1, and also relates to communication, commitment and competence – three of the 6 Cs. These require you to be open to new experiences while recognising limitations to your knowledge and taking the necessary action to resolve the limitation. Thus, life-long learning comes with an individual responsibility to actively pursue learning as well as being part of your preparation programme. Life-long learning differs from life-long education in that learning is about developing your understanding across the spectrum of your life, whereas education might be assumed to refer to the ways these ideas might be taught (Jarvis, 2010).

What is life-deep learning?

Life-long learning in a life-wide sense invites an approach to learning that includes how others have influenced you (West et al., 2007). In other words, you could say that life-long and life-wide learning take place within a context of life-deep learning. Banks et al. (2007) suggest that life-deep learning includes moral, ethical, spiritual and social values that guide what we believe, how we act, and how we view ourselves and others. These authors suggest that, as humans, we construct our lives around symbols. Family life is instrumental in our learning, teaches us to understand symbols of communication, and provides us with a multitude of skills and tasks. The learning available to the family members does, however, take place according to our specific family *culture* and tradition. We can understand the powerful nature of this learning when we are confronted with other cultural beliefs and habits, for example, when we travel abroad. We will come back to this idea called *cultural competency* later in this book. You can see how life-long aspects of learning relate to whom you are within your relationships with people, which is linked to the culture you have grown up in, your history, hopes and ideas, as well as your goals. For example, how does your experience of learning in its widest sense influence your approaches to ongoing learning? This might relate to the way feelings produced by past learning experiences are taken forward and how they influence your engagement with further learning. A good example of this is the 'mental block' some students experience when being assessed on their numeracy proficiency, which is often related to their earlier school experience.

The challenges of learning to understand communication symbols can clearly be seen in how we sometimes have difficulty in interpreting verbal and non-verbal communication and is also the reason that virtual communication media such as email, Twitter, etc.

can easily be misunderstood. We learn language and behavioural symbols in relation to roles such as child, parent, pupil or student, and these are possibly very different to the role of a healthcare professional. You might already have seen that there are different expectations of you, as a student or as a student nurse, to previous expectations you may have had.

Activity 2.2   Looking for symbols

Please take a few minutes to think of any different expectations with regard to your language or behaviour that you might have noticed since starting the nursing programme. Write these down and then cluster them according to whether you think the language or behaviour symbol is a professional expectation or whether they are peer expectations due to you being in a new group.

As this activity is based on your own experiences, there is no outline answer at the end of the chapter.

Looking back at what we've covered so far in this chapter, it is clear that we are not uni-dimensional but complex individuals whose learning is influenced by multiple factors. Although healthcare often draws on knowledge relating to the body there are many more areas where, as nurses, we need to stay abreast of developments. Think back to the concerns raised in Chapter 1 about how the body is viewed, and to the outcome skills at the start of this chapter relating to healthcare organisation and structures. As healthcare becomes more complex, less compassionate and more impersonal, staff members need to take a more holistic view that considers emotional and social dimensions when working with people (Howatson-Jones and Thurgate, 2014). Learning involves social elements through our interactions, emotional aspects perceived by how we feel about things and cognitive parts representing our thinking (Illeris, 2009). These all have an influence on our sense of self and our learning. Life-long learning encompasses a number of dimensions that interconnect according to your intentions and opportunities, as illustrated in Figure 2.1.

As suggested in Figure 2.1, formal learning is usually directed towards a learning outcome. For example, your nursing programme is based on a curriculum, verified by the regulatory body, covering what you need to know to work as a registered nurse. The outcome to the programme is being able to function at a specific level as a registered nurse at the end of the programme. Incidental learning occurs alongside the formal learning activities and is influenced by the quality of these activities and experiences. Informal (life-wide) learning relates to the discussions you may have with your peers

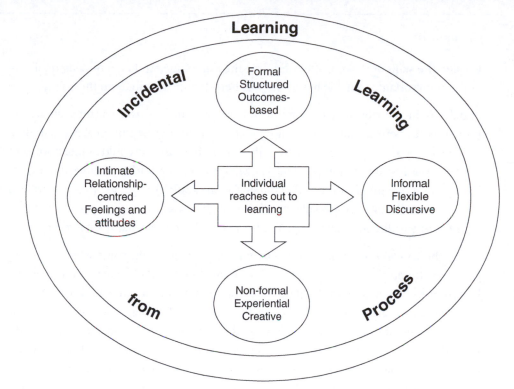

Figure 2.1 Some dimensions of learning

and patients, which also help to develop your thinking and knowledge. Experiential (life-long) learning relates to what you learn from dealing with different situations. Relationship-centred (life-deep) learning is about how you learn to manage attitudes and feelings within your encounters with others.

As an individual, we are at the centre of our learning. It is up to us whether we actually engage with it and discern what we have learned. How we integrate different ways of learning is, in itself, another form of learning and a major part of life-long learning. In order to do this, we need to reflect on our learning, build on what we already know, make possible connections between different forms of learning and consider our development. Consider the case study below involving Shuki's integration of her learning in order to identify how integrated reflection might contribute to further learning.

Case study: Shuki's integration of her learning

Shuki came from an Indian family where she was the middle child of five siblings. As both her parents worked, she had often helped with her siblings and consequently

(Continued)

(Continued)

learned the skills of looking after herself at the same time. To her, a nursing qualification was important to enable her to support herself and contribute to the family.

Shuki was in the first year of her nursing programme and was learning about the human body, person-centred nursing practice and her developing professional identity. She enjoyed the practical aspects of the course because she could connect some of what she was learning to her previous knowledge of caring for her siblings in terms of hygiene and bathing, feeding and elimination. Shuki did find some of the theoretical elements hard to grasp, especially the clinical science sessions, which seemed so full of jargon that she did not really understand. Shuki reflected on what she could do.

When she thought about it, Shuki equated the problem to learning a different language. At home she spoke an Indian dialect and English, and remembered how she had found it easier to learn English from her friends. Maybe she could draw on her bilingual experiences to help her learn this scientific language. Shuki decided this would be easier if she could share this with others and so asked some of her class if they wanted to form a revision group. They agreed to meet, on an informal basis, before class on Thursday for two hours, to go over what they had learned in the previous session and fill in the gaps. Some of the revision group had other learning needs and one student, Michael, volunteered to summarise their learning into an ongoing revision document for them all to use. Michael checked the accuracy of the document with the module tutor who was impressed by the group's initiative.

Shuki was surprised and pleased at her success in arranging this group. When she reflected on this she also recognised that some of her experiences of managing herself were also instrumental in this organisation and design of her learning and developing assertiveness. By drawing together different threads of her learning she was also able to contribute to her further learning.

Having read this case study, you might have started to reflect on your own life-long learning and how different aspects might connect to make something new. Try to relate this exercise back to Activity 2.2 and analyse what this might mean for you. Undertaking Activity 2.3 offers you an opportunity to think about your life-long learning and reach some conclusions.

Activity 2.3   Reflection

Think about your learning since you started your nursing programme. If you are in your first year of the programme, you might want to consider the following questions:

- How has my view of nursing changed and why?
- What skills have I learned?
- How has my identity changed?
- How have my values changed?

If you are further on in the programme you might want to think about the following:

- What areas of my knowledge have changed and why?
- What areas of my knowledge do I need to develop further and why?

If you are an experienced practitioner, you might want to think about the following.

- What changes have happened in healthcare since I started in my practitioner role?
- What knowledge change has this required from me?
- How did I develop this knowledge?
- How have I developed my evidence base?
- What further goals do I have for my learning?

There is some guidance about this activity at the end of the chapter.

When completing this activity, you might have considered different contexts and ways in which you increased your knowledge and evidence base during your nurse preparation programme and over time. We now proceed to look at some contexts in which learning takes place.

Contexts in which learning takes place

The theoretical learning that you undertake in university provides you with the necessary background information to inform your practice, just as your practice can help you to make sense of the theory you've learned, but can also inform theory when something new is identified, for example, in the way that a patient responds to the interventions in which you are involved. Your placements are another context for learning from the experiences you have there. Patients are all different, as are the contexts in which they are nursed. Each of these experiences offers an opportunity for learning. So, with so many scenarios contained within each clinical shift, one could argue that it is not possible, as some students state, not to be able to learn anything in a particular placement area. It is so important to be aware of learning opportunities that arise and be proactive in using them to your advantage.

Learning, whether undertaken in university or in practice, can also be shared with others. Learning as a group is a valuable way of turning ideas into articulated thinking, as was illustrated in Shuki's case study. The process of explaining something to someone else shows us what we really understand about an issue and, at the same time, the feedback from others opens the possibilities of further thinking to develop understanding. The virtual world may provide another avenue for expanding our ideas and learning when others are not immediately available to converse or share ideas with.

The virtual world can be both a public and a private space for learning, for example, virtual learning environment (VLE) discussion boards may be viewed by many course participants and are public. Contributions may, correspondingly, be less spontaneous and more thought through before being placed in such a public domain, because of possible concerns with and anticipation of others' reactions (Kozlowski, 2002). In this context it is sometimes harder to acknowledge unfinished thinking. Nevertheless, electronic resources also provide opportunities for learning that are individually focused. For example, you can look up the action of a particular drug or disease process, or identify the latest research underpinning a particular nursing intervention. This learning can be accessed and completed in private and at your own pace.

There may be times when you are too shy to ask, and it may be tempting to rely solely on virtual sources for information that do not expose you to the scrutiny of others but, having said that, do not underestimate the importance of testing your ideas with educators or peers. Only through doing this can you establish whether you are thinking along the correct lines. However, it is also important to remember that not all electronic sources or sites are credible, and some information may be biased. It is important to make sure that such learning is related to some framework for learning to help you stay focused. You will also need to have access to reliable guidance to help evaluate what you have found in order to avoid mistakes. An example might be looking something up and then discussing this further with your practice supervisor or course tutor. In the case study about Shuki above, the revision guide created by the group was checked with the module tutor by Michael, for accuracy. This not only helps to avoid mistakes, but may also help to share learning that is beneficial with others.

When trying anything for the first time there is an element of learning from the mistakes you might make. Mistakes can be a valuable way of learning when you reflect on what went wrong, analyse the processes that led to the mistake and consider what you can do to avoid making the same mistake again. Taking responsibility for what has gone wrong enables new ideas to develop (Ranse and Grealish, 2007; Rogers and Freiberg, 1994). Mistakes, although unpleasant in their possible consequences and challenges to self-esteem, also provide emotional learning about how to deal with anxiety and disappointment, and how to move on in a positive way. Support for such learning may come from family members or close peers, as well as through the encouragement of colleagues. Nevertheless, this requires time and motivation to really reflect on what has been learned. To help you understand some of these points relating to learning from mistakes, please consider Scenario 2.2 and then complete Activity 2.4.

Scenario 2.2: Kevin's mistake

Kevin was working in a nursing home and was in the first year of his nursing programme. He had been working in the home for two weeks and was starting to get to know the people and processes. Today Kevin was looking after Jim. Jim had had a urinary accident in his carpeted room and Kevin went to inform his practice supervisor, Briony, to find out what to do because Kevin assumed this would be dealt with differently to what he would do in his own home. Briony told Kevin he would need to use a spillage kit to remove the urine from the carpet and she would join him shortly, but first needed to finish giving her residents their drugs.

Kevin found the spillage kit and, wanting to appear helpful and, because the instructions appeared straightforward, proceeded to start using the kit before Briony joined him. On entering the room Briony found Kevin coughing with his eyes streaming. She immediately helped him to wash his eyes out and told him to go off duty to A&E to get himself checked out. Unbeknown to Briony, Kevin sat in the staff room downstairs for half an hour until she went off duty and as he felt better he went back upstairs to complete his hours.

The next day when Kevin came on duty Briony asked him what the A&E staff had said. Kevin replied that he had not gone to A&E. Briony was angry about this but managed to stay calm. When she and Kevin had completed their work, she asked Kevin to come into the seminar room with her to discuss the episode and complete a statement.

Activity 2.4 Reflection

* What are the significant aspects of this scenario and why?
* What questions might Briony have for Kevin?
* Why is it important for Kevin to reflect on the actions/inactions that he undertook?
* Which of the 6 Cs are relevant in the scenario and why?

If you are a student you might want to reflect on a situation where you, perhaps, tried resolve a situation that did not go entirely to plan. If you are an experienced practitioner think about what you want to consider as the practice supervisor.

There are outline answers to these questions at the end of the chapter.

Scenario 2.2 may have identified some of the difficulties involved for the novice practitioner in trying to fit into a new environment and team. It might also have highlighted some problems that could arise from inaction. Both are contexts of learning and we need to be able to reconcile the formal and the less formal. We now proceed to consider some features of formal and less formal ways of learning.

Features of learning in formal and less formal ways

Features of formal learning involve codifying information into our thinking (Eraut, 2001). What this means is that the information is often already offered in the form of categories and theories, which we embed in our thinking according to particular required outcomes. This may make concepts easier to grasp, but at the same time might also inhibit the development of different interpretations. Reflecting on formal learning can help to negate such effects by opening up alternative views. Consider some features in your formal learning by completing Activity 2.5.

Activity 2.5   Critical thinking

Think about a recent class you attended as part of your nurse preparation programme. What features of learning can you identify by considering the following questions:

- How did the lesson start?
- What were you asked to do during the lesson?
- How did the lesson finish?
- What did you learn?
- Did you do anything further to aid your learning after the lesson and, if so, what did you do?

If you are an experienced practitioner consider a recent continuing professional development (CPD) session.

There is an outline answer to this activity at the end of the chapter.

Formal learning often provides some initial knowledge for practice and is often the start of the process of professional learning. However, sharing experiences with peers in a less formal way is an important feature of professional learning. When informally sharing experiences, different interpretations, based on subjective experiences, may be offered and explored, allowing debate and reconsideration of the conclusions that might be reached. The feature of this learning is its evolving and discursive nature, which means that it is flexible and responsive, but therefore it can be harder to quantify this form of evidence. Personal learning can help support professional practice and is another feature of less formal ways of learning through reworking personal knowledge within the professional setting. An example might be having the ability to speak another language and using this to translate in the professional setting. Integration of personal and professional learning supports a holistic approach to health and social care. Please consider some features of your less formal learning by completing Activity 2.6.

Activity 2.6   Critical thinking

Think about a recent discussion you had in practice. What features of learning can you identify by examining the following?

- What prompted the discussion?
- What were the key arguments made?
- What was the outcome of the discussion?
- What did you learn?
- Did you do anything further to aid your learning?

There is an outline answer to this activity at the end of the chapter.

Within Activity 2.5 and Activity 2.6 you will have had an opportunity to compare and contrast different forms of learning. We now proceed to look at types of knowledge and ways of knowing that are relevant to the healthcare practitioner.

Types of knowledge and ways of knowing

Theories and protocols – what Eraut (2001) calls propositional knowledge – are important for identifying what knowledge is expected of the professional learner. Examples include theories of communication and psychological processing, how the human body works, disease effects, infection control and much more. Protocols, such as NICE (National Institute for Health and Care Excellence) guidelines, relate to identification of what is required within a particular situation such as assessment procedures, what to do when someone suffers a stroke or cardiac arrest, or how to prepare somebody for an operation. These constitute professional knowledge and should reflect best practice standards. In other words, these would be professional ways of knowing that relate to the meaning that a professional derives from a situation through experience and from applying theory and evidence to practice.

Practical knowledge relates to knowing how to do things and developing the skills required to carry them out. This knowledge is part of the *professional craft* (Titchen et al., 2004, p108).

Aesthetic knowing

Personal knowledge comes from the *life-world* of individuals (Jarvis, 2006). This means that it comes from their background, culture, with whom they interact and the activities in which they are involved. It also relates to how individuals see themselves and others. Personal knowledge develops from reflecting on events and making sense of situations and is illustrated in Figure 2.1 as 'incidental knowledge from process'. Over time, layers of experience may filter into the unconscious and re-emerge later as intuitive knowing. The following short case study is offered as an example of how the different types of knowledge and knowing may all interlink in your practice of healthcare.

Case study: Suzy's day

Suzy was in her last year of the nursing programme. She was working in an *oncology* setting, which she enjoyed. There were clear guidelines for when patients were due to have particular treatments, and Suzy had spent today discussing some of these with her practice supervisor, Ben, in order to gain a better understanding. Ben had first explored Suzy's knowledge of the relevant clinical science relating to various types of cancers, in particular the cell development cycle and how this was important to determine treatment phases.

The discussion between Suzy and Ben then moved forward to her assessment, which was due soon. Suzy identified that many of the patients required regular blood tests and, although Suzy had been trained in *venepuncture* in her previous role as a healthcare assistant (HCA), she understood that she was not allowed to undertake this in her current role as a student because of differences in responsibility and accountability. Ben highlighted, however, that Suzy was always ready with the required equipment when other nurses needed to take a sample, which they valued. She had also been quick to identify *phlebitis* in a patient, which was undoubtedly due to her previous experience.

Ben asked Suzy to reflect on why she enjoyed working in this particular setting and what she thought she had learned. When thinking about this, Suzy identified that dignity, respect and compassion were important values for her. Supporting people with cancer was fulfilling for her because of the opportunity to really listen and attend to someone else's situation, because she was not able to be involved in some of the treatments. From this she had learned what therapeutic relationship and communication might actually mean in practice and not just as an abstract idea. Suzy told Ben that reflection on this placement had enabled her to bring the abstract idea of the 6 Cs to life through the identification of her values and the depth of communication she had practised. She felt, because she had 'lived' this learning, it would stay with her.

Through reading the case study you may have noted how professional, practical and personal knowledge may be integrated in a typical day. The role of reflection in achieving this is paramount. We finish this chapter by highlighting how learning is related to reflection.

Learning and reflection

Processes of learning can carry mixed emotions which can get in the way of learning experiences, because of anxiety that might be aroused. Learning reams of facts also does not embed understanding or application of learning. In order to transform learning into something that you can apply in different situations with different people and at different times, reflection on learning is required to enable examination of what has actually been learned. It is through reflection that connections can be made for:

- life-wide and life-long learning;
- learning and life-deep learning;
- different types of learning;
- different types of knowledge and knowing;
- the evidence base being used;
- how to deal with emotions;
- what values and beliefs are developing;
- what alternatives are available;
- what the likely outcomes are;
- what nursing is.

Chapter summary

This chapter started to examine some of the issues listed above and offers a variety of opportunities to make some of these connections through the case studies, activities and scenarios provided. By undertaking the activities, it has been possible for you to apply some of the ideas around life-wide, life-long and life-deep learning in different settings and at different stages of the nurse preparation programme. This is a crucial part of continuing life-long learning as set out in the NMC's *Standards of Proficiency for Registered Nurses* (NMC, 2018a) at the start of the chapter, in order to meet the challenges of healthcare evolving and changing. How to explore life-wide learning in greater depth is the subject of Chapter 3.

Activities and scenarios: Brief outline answers

Activity 2.1 Critical thinking (page 32)

Your answer might have included:

- how to communicate in different groups;

- how to communicate with different people or in different situations;
- developing friendships;
- using the internet to find information, writing up notes, reading;
- learning to drive, swim, play a sport;
- learning to cook, manage finance, become a parent;
- learning to problem solve.

As indicated when the activity was introduced, you might find it helpful to develop a visual map of all your learning first and then group various categories together.

Activity 2.3 Reflection (pages 36–7)

If you are a novice practitioner in your first year, your answer might have considered:

- nursing is hard work and emotionally challenging;
- skills learned in the first year include recording nursing observations such as temperature, pulse, respiration, and blood pressure and oxygen saturations, and undertaking urinalysis, bed bathing, simple wound care, administering injections, checking medications with the practice supervisor and caring for urinary catheters;
- identity changes might include becoming more assertive and confident.

If you are further on in your nurse preparation programme, you might have thought about:

- having more knowledge about how clinical science applies in practice;
- a need to develop wider knowledge of pharmacology and pathophysiology in order to understand treatment options.

If you are an experienced practitioner, you might have thought about:

- increasing use of technology in nursing observations and interventions;
- the move to an all-graduate profession for nursing;
- returning to further formal academic study;
- investigating new opportunities and knowledge requirements in nursing.

Activity 2.4 Reflection on Kevin's mistake (page 39)

The significant aspects of Scenario 2.2 are Kevin not following instructions and listening to his practice supervisor, and trying to do things on his own before he has been given the relevant information. It is important when new to any environment to be oriented to the correct processes and procedures, and to accept supervision as an important support rather than a sign of weakness. By not following his practice supervisor's instructions, Kevin has put patients and himself at risk through poor infection control procedure, and not looking after his own health and safety. The questions Briony might have discussed with Kevin in the seminar room could have included why he did not wait for her before starting to use the spillage kit and why he did not get himself checked in A&E. Briony could then use Kevin's answers as teaching aids to demonstrate how using her support could provide more positive outcomes. Briony might ask Kevin to write a reflection about this for her and his personal tutor to consolidate his learning from this.

Kevin's best intentions should not be overlooked because it is important to show initiative, but also to understand the potential risks. Care, communication and commitment may have been three of the 6 Cs motivating Kevin to undertake the action he did. His desire to care for Jim and his living environment and commitment to his role of a nurse, not wanting to unduly burden Briony, and to show that he was able to use his own initiative and that he was not above doing 'menial' tasks. Communication is possibly a key point to consider – the written instructions on the spillage kit appearing quite straightforward, but without adequate warning of potential dangers which, otherwise, could have alerted Kevin to the risks. Briony, assuming that Kevin would implicitly understand that she was not suggesting he wait because of the seeming 'simplicity' of the task at hand, but rather that he wait because it was a more complex and risk-laden procedure. This could be a point of reflection for Briony, namely to reflect on how she communicates a potentially hazardous activity. As part of this exercise, it is recommended that you consult the NMC's Code (2018b). Kevin's actions, although well intended, placed Briony in a difficult position because she could be seen to have breached different areas of the Code such as *Practise effectively* (item 7.4) which states that a nurse should check people's understanding to minimise misunderstanding and mistakes. Similarly, Kevin might have put the resident, Jim, at risk from the fumes, which could have breached item 8.5. It is, therefore, important to realise that risk assessment not only concerns service users, but applies also to staff being safe at work, and can have far-reaching effects if not adhered to.

As a student you might want to reflect on:

- how you set boundaries and how you assess the risk of what you do;
- what makes you want to try things for yourself, e.g. not wanting to make demands on your practice supervisor, you feel restricted in your development by not being able to make decisions yourself, or you are aware of your learning style;
- how clear you have been in discussing your plans for the placement – in other words, have you been proactive in setting your learning outcomes, have you discussed your learning style with your practice supervisor and which style of support works for you, etc.?
- if you find you're unable to approach your practice supervisor openly, why is this and what action can you take to improve the relationship, etc.?

As an experienced practitioner thinking as a practice supervisor you might consider:

- how to maintain a supportive learning relationship while correcting practice;
- how to construct feedback to support safe and effective practice;
- the need to involve university representatives;
- how to act on the learning results.

Activity 2.5 Critical thinking (page 40)

Your answer might have identified that the lesson started with the learning objectives of what you were expected to learn. You might have been asked to discuss some of the concepts in smaller groups and apply these to practice scenarios. The lesson might have finished by summarising the main points. You might have identified that you remembered some of the key points and might have undertaken some further reading of your notes. You could also have undertaken self-study to clarify terminology or concepts you did not fully understand, or you may have created a glossary of terms to which you can refer.

As an experienced practitioner thinking about a CPD session, you might have considered how the lesson started by enquiring about your present knowledge of the topic. During the session you are likely to have discussed application to your practice, in small groups. The session could have finished with a summary of the key points and guidance on directed study. You might have tried to fit in the directed study around your workload and expanded your learning through further discussion with work colleagues. You could have used the insights and knowledge gained from the session to critically consider the strengths and weaknesses in your area of work.

Activity 2.6 Critical thinking (page 41)

Your answer might have identified that a patient problem stimulated the discussion. Key points of this discussion are likely to have included some background information about the problem, who should be involved and possible solutions. The outcome is likely to have been an agreement on the solution to be implemented. Perhaps you thought about the intervention and considered whether alternatives may have been more appropriate. You could also have wondered on what evidence the decision for the intervention was based. You might have identified learning about decision-making, team working and problem solving. You might have reflected on this further afterwards. Have you noticed that it seems more natural to reflect on situations that are based on relationships?

The aspects of learning and reflection identified in this activity will possibly seem quite logical and obvious. Hopefully they are, but the objective of this is to help you become aware of the importance of these activities and to remind you that this seemingly obvious activity is part of professional practice and is included in the NMC's Code (2018b).

Further reading

Mason-Whitehead, E and Mason, T (2008) *Study Skills for Nurses*, 2nd edn. Los Angeles, CA: Sage.

This book has a useful section on life-long learning which includes the formal and less formal. It also relates life-long learning to continuing career development when the nurse preparation programme has been completed.

Thomas, C (2019) Sources of knowledge for evidence-based care. In P Ellis, ed., *Evidence-based Practice in Nursing*, 4th edn. London: Sage, Chapter 2.

Clear and concise guide on how to search for and access relevant evidence via electronic information sources and digital media.

Chapter 3 Autobiographical reflection and learning

Chapter aims

After reading this chapter you will be able to:

- consider how reflection integrates the personal with the professional, drawing on experiences from all areas of life;
- complete a life story construction exercise;
- creatively explore your experiences by reflecting on your life story;
- integrate reflection and learning with a sense of developing values and a developing identity;
- reflect on aspects of your life that may also reveal societal issues.

Introduction

Scenario 3.1: Lizzie's autobiographical experience

Lizzie came from a large family. She had three older and two younger siblings. Her parents both worked. Her older brothers had left home and her sister, who was in her late teens, was intent on pursuing her own social life. One night, when she was 16, Lizzie offered to stay with her younger siblings so that her parents could go out for a meal to celebrate her mother's birthday. Her younger brother and sister were 12 and 8, respectively, at the time, so it was not too much of a hardship to keep an eye on them.

While playing an electronic game with her brother, Lizzie noticed that her sister Amy was looking very tired and becoming distressed with the flashing lights and loud noises from the game. She suggested that Amy might be better going to bed. When she went to say goodnight to Amy she noticed that she looked very pale. Amy pulled up her pyjama top and showed Lizzie a collection of spots on her abdomen. Lizzie remembered an advertisement for the warning signs of meningitis that she had seen on the television. She got a glass and rolled it over the spots. They did not fade. She also noted that, earlier, Amy had been avoiding the lights and noises of the game. Lizzie took action, calling her parents and an ambulance. It was later confirmed that Amy did indeed have meningitis and that Lizzie's vigilance had ensured she received treatment early. Her parents were full of praise. Lizzie felt emotionally confused, happy that her sister was recovering, but also guilty that she had not noticed earlier.

A few years later, no one was surprised that Lizzie chose to become a children's nurse. When she was writing her statement for consideration for entry to the programme, Lizzie reflected on this episode in order to identify some of her attributes. She concluded that she had the observational and decision-making skills required of a nurse, but also considered that this episode had taught her that there were emotional consequences to caring work.

As a student nurse, Lizzie has reflected further on how the emotional residue from caring work may be different when dealing with situations personally or professionally. She has used her autobiographical experience to develop discussion with her peers about the observation of symptoms and disease as well as the emotional consequences of critical incidents. Through sharing this story, she has come to a better understanding of herself as a capable and caring person who copes well in critical situations, but who also requires emotional support to work through her thinking.

This chapter has started with an example scenario to help illustrate how your life story can help student nurses make sense of their capabilities and progress. You will have entered into the nursing programme with a variety of experiences. These will influence your perception and experience of yourself, of others and of practice. In Scenario 3.1

Lizzie's capabilities are affirmed, but through further reflection she has been able to identify areas she can develop more. Developing reflective insight is an important starting point for any person entering a caring profession, and particularly nursing. Such insight explains why we react and think in certain ways, what resources in the form of family and friends and personal knowledge are available to us, and what the possibilities might be for development and change.

When talking about life stories we are referring to our autobiographies. In other words, how do our family, school, work and social experiences and formal learning make us who we are, and influence how we think, how we react, our norms and values and our ambitions. As you can imagine, reflecting on these areas of our lives can sometimes be challenging, painful or confrontational but, at the same time, enriching and exciting. To do this effectively, it takes courage and commitment – two of the 6 Cs. The point being made here is that we cannot, in effect, separate the personal and the professional – the two are inextricably linked and any change in one will, automatically, result in a change to the other. Looking at Lizzie's example in Scenario 3.1, we can see that the emotional baggage she carried from the experience with her younger sister has made her more attuned to the emotional risks associated with caring for children. This insight into her own response seems to motivate her to care for peers and colleagues by 'warning' them of the pitfalls. Had she not had this personal experience, it is possible that she would have been unaware of potential emotional risks to her and her colleagues. Conversely, we could argue that there is a possibility that Lizzie could become more extreme in her perception of emotional risk and become overburdened through an inability to filter her experiences.

As indicated, this chapter introduces the idea of autobiographical reflection as a way to advance nursing knowledge in different ways. It will first define what autobiographical reflection is before proceeding to consider how to integrate personal and professional experience, and the importance of doing so. You will be invited to construct your own autobiography with guidance on the key points for inclusion in the construction. This is followed by further guidance on how to examine and reflect on your autobiography. The chapter ends by looking at how societal issues may be given meaning through subjective experience.

What is autobiographical reflection?

As people progress through life they begin to develop a life history. This history, just like any other, charts the timeline of events and changes that have come about. It also includes motives for particular actions, how situations have been shaped, how the individual has been shaped by events and their aspirations for the future. From the experiences that individuals have in their lives, personal knowledge develops. Experiences may be very diverse, because they result from the ways in which we come into contact with the world and make sense of it through interacting with it (Boud and Miller, 1996). This resonates with Bhabha's (2004) work in which he describes a 'third space'. This arises from one individual connecting with another or a group and, through shared experiences and perceptions, a hybrid way of perceiving the world is created. For example, going to school exposes an individual to many different people and types of learning. Others' reactions to efforts made at interacting and understanding provide feedback that is internalised as knowledge of personal ability. Read Scenario 3.2 about Callum's biographical account of school to identify what learning he might have taken forward from this experience.

Scenario 3.2: Callum's biographical account of school

Callum went to a private secondary school. He had struggled with learning at primary school and his parents decided that the smaller class sizes and greater individual attention offered by private education might benefit him. Callum was dyslexic, struggled with learning, and was often made fun of by his peers and called 'stupid' in class. However, Callum excelled at sport, particularly rugby where he demonstrated good leadership qualities as team captain. The nature of the game meant that players got injured and Callum would help to provide assistance because he had taken a first aid course that he enjoyed because of its practical nature which he found easy to understand. After leaving school Callum went into nursing because of the practical nature of the work and before it required university-based study.

After qualifying as a nurse Callum completed mainly clinically practical courses relating to his nursing work. He progressed some way in his career but realised that in order to go further he would need to complete formal study, because nursing education, including continuing professional development, was now located within universities. Callum worked with a supervisor who came into his practice area from the university to help him write a reflective account of different learning he had achieved over the years, in order to submit in a portfolio of evidence. This attracted academic credits equivalent to a diploma.

Callum really enjoyed undertaking this reflective work. It suited his *learning style* and his supervisor offered continual feedback so that his final portfolio was presentable and relatively error free. Callum achieved a mark of 55 per cent and felt encouraged to continue on to the degree.

Activity 3.1   Reflection

- What learning is Callum taking forward from school?
- What learning is Callum taking forward from his portfolio study experience?

There is an outline answer to this activity at the end of the chapter.

Scenario 3.2 identifies that experiences of learning can be both positive and challenging. Horsdal (2012, p25) suggests that the way we use our senses and communicate affects the development of our 'social brain'. Sharing our experiences with an empathetic listener, such as Callum did with his supervisor, means that we can retrace our paths in a supported way and consequently learn from our experiences. In such a way experiences can be transformed through autobiographical reflection. An autobiography turns these experiences into an account of what has been lived through and the meaning that has been attached to this as part of a personal history. Autobiography reviews individual experiences within the life history and reflection scrutinises links between them to explore how the past might be influencing the present. In doing so, it finds creative ways to address situations and problems by drawing on personal knowledge that has come from a personal history. In this way autobiographical reflection helps to make sense of past experiences within an individual life history and what might be being taken forward, raising the possibility of change. This will also be the case for professional experiences, certainly at the start of your professional career. The only reference upon which to reflect is our personal experience. As we build our professional experience, so we have more 'professional landmarks' to reflect on and, in time, we may feel that our 'professional values' differ from our 'personal values'. This is an interesting phenomenon which is why continual reflection on and awareness of how we are developing is so important. Not doing this can lead to alienation from yourself and those close to you. Just think for a moment of the things you experience in your first placement of your nursing programme; often you see and experience more challenging and emotional situations than some people experience in their entire lives. Reflection on your experiences – good and bad – helps you develop resilience and cope more effectively with things that cross your professional and personal paths.

We do not always pay attention to the experiences that we come into contact with and therefore may not recognise their value in terms of what has been learned and what can be translated into different circumstances and situations. Equally, there may be times when it feels like we have reached an impasse by perhaps becoming too overwhelmed by the situation to be able to move forward. For example, learning anatomy and physiology can be difficult for some people and yet these are integral parts of nursing knowledge. If you have artistic attributes, these could potentially play a part in how you perceive things and possibly respond to them. You may be more drawn to the art of nursing than perhaps the science. Understanding this is a first step to dealing with potential difficulties that might arise in learning the language and structure of scientific theories.

So, we see that autobiographical reflection is not limited to clinical experiences or negative experiences; we also learn that all experiences can be used to learn from. It is a way of making sense of what is happening, set within the context of a person's life. By focusing attention on that person's life history we can identify how people can renegotiate a position and deal with the challenge they are facing (Horsdal, 2007). This renegotiation is called 'agency', and by this individuals can take control of their lives. Individuals use their life resources to construct strategies for developing and dealing with change (West et al., 2007). Therefore, in the example of the artistic student nurse, it might be that revision notes using colour and drawing is one way to surmount an obstacle to understanding scientific concepts. Although there have been numerous definitions and descriptions of reflection, in essence they can be related back to work by Boud et al. (1985, p19), indicating that reflection, in the first instance, requires:

- returning to experience;
- attending to feelings;
- re-evaluating experience;
- planning change.

This is not dissimilar to the reflective cycle suggested by Barksby et al. (2015, p22). In this model, the authors recommend seven stages in the reflective cycle which clearly mirror Boud et al. (1985):

R – RECALL (the events);

E – EXAMINE (your responses);

F – (acknowledge) FEELINGS;

L – LEARN (from the experience);

E – EXPLORE (options);

C – CREATE (a plan of action);

T – (set) TIMESCALE.

Activity 3.2 Reflection

Look back at Scenario 3.2 (Callum's biographical account of school and learning as a nurse) and consider the following.

- What meaning do you think he has attached to his experiences?
- What creative ways might he find to help his learning?

There is an outline answer to this activity at the end of the chapter.

Autobiographical reflection explores personal learning in how the past is combined with perceptions of sensations within the present (Jarvis, 2007). Such reflection involves thinking about how, in the first instance, to construct the autobiographical account in terms of what to include, what seems relevant in the present moment and why. For example, it can be helpful to gather autobiographical experiences of learning – what Dominice (2000) calls *writing an educational biography* – in order to develop an understanding of personal learning processes via reflecting on diverse learning experiences through the life history. Such autobiographical reflection looks at learning in its widest sense of formal and informal experience. This can be a very valuable exercise in terms of both academic and practice learning. It can be challenging when you do not receive the mark you had anticipated for an assignment or you are given points to improve on by your practice supervisor. It is worth reflecting on how you receive this information: do you accept it graciously, possibly asking for further clarification? Or do you become defensive, feel embarrassed or feel that you are a failure? These are exactly the valuable points to reflect on – why do you feel this way? Is it your 'voice' or is it the 'voice' of a teacher at secondary school? Is what the teacher then said still valid? You are, after all, older, have more life experience and are in a very different situation. This is a strong reflective topic. So often nursing students become paralysed at the thought of numeracy, research or science-related subjects when, on further exploration, one finds that they have had a challenging or traumatic experience in school – perhaps failing an exam or feeling humiliated in front of their peers. It is helpful to understand why you think or are afraid that this will happen again and, possibly more importantly, why you think that your reaction will be the same. These are all excellent topics for reflection.

Apply consideration of autobiographical experience to your own life by completing Activity 3.3.

Activity 3.3 Critical thinking

Spend a little time thinking of a particular story from your life history – this could be from your personal or professional experience – and write it down. Please then answer the following questions:

- What made you think of that story?
- What feelings does the story bring back for you and why?
- Whose 'voices' appear in the story and what are your relationships and connections with them?
- What has changed between then and now, how has it changed and why might that be?
- Can you think of ways in which writing your autobiography might help develop your learning in terms of this story?

There is some guidance on this activity at the end of the chapter.

Autobiographical reflection also requires acknowledging how we feel about the past, and this may be difficult in terms of the emotional aspects that might appear or resurface. Nevertheless, being able to deal with your own emotions is one of the essential skills associated with being a nurse. The ability to acknowledge feelings and recognise what stimulates them, and why, is also a way of recognising our own humanity; this is an important aspect when entering a caring profession. This was emphasised in Chapter 1, in the story about Heather in Scenario 1.1, who worked in a learning disability community placement and highlighted uncaring behaviours that she felt did not recognise the humanity of others, interpreting these as possible reasons for care failings. Remaining detached can be another way of coping, by suppressing feelings from past situations that are still active within the present. Cultural values are another rich stream that can also be explored through autobiographical reflection and is looked at in more detail in Chapter 6.

Having explored what autobiographical reflection is, and having provided a few examples, we now move on to consider in more detail how personal and professional experience might be integrated.

Integrating personal and professional experience

Personal experience is a rich resource that may not always be seen as relevant to professional life, or professional experience. Nevertheless, as we've already mentioned, the skills and knowledge developed within personal experience are the foundation from which individuals develop their professional identity and skills. For example, some of the roles that people inhabit within their lives, such as being a parent, a member of a committee or community group, a community group leader, an activity teacher and so on, bring valuable experiences that integrate with professional experience, to advance knowledge and practice in different ways, thereby enhancing knowledge and skills. Completing Activity 3.4 will help you to identify what different roles and experiences you can bring to that of being a (student) nurse.

Activity 3.4   Reflection

Take some time at this point to consider what roles you occupy in your personal life and the different activities you are involved in. Make a list of these – it is preferable to write the things down that you are requested to do because this will make them more tangible. You might be thinking of roles such as artist, activist, volunteer, carer, but these examples are not exhaustive and there are many others that could bring equally valuable experience. Bear in mind that the knowledge derived from the roles is dependent on length of time you have been in the role, which transferable skills you have learned, and your degree of confidence to show and articulate your experiences.

Now consider how these roles might integrate with your professional life. Spend a little time reflecting on the following questions. You might find this easier for yourself if you try to focus on one role at a time and work through all the questions before moving on to the next one.

- What knowledge is used in fulfilling the role? Where did you get this knowledge? Were you aware that you were learning this role? If so, provide some detail on this experience.
- Are any particular skills involved and, if so, what are they? How did you learn the skills? Were you aware of this learning? If so, provide some detail on this experience.
- How might these skills be translated into different situations? In other words, think of examples where you have been able to use things that you've learned in one situation in a completely different situation.
- Where are there connections with the professional role?

As this activity is based on your own experiences, there is no outline answer at the end of the chapter.

Having completed Activity 3.4, you should now have a clearer idea of where to direct your reflection. Integrating personal and professional experience involves reflecting on what each contributes and how they may relate to each other. It is worthwhile remembering that both personal and professional experiences feed into one result – you. As previously mentioned, a change in one will automatically impact on the other. It is within integration that knowledge can be brought together as a whole or synthesised in more creative ways. For example, some of the knowledge developed through the parenting role is likely to include lifespan development, disease management, communication and negotiation, leadership, organisation, nutrition, first aid and learning. Integration involves connecting this with what is learned through your professional role and through reflecting imaginatively, identifying possibilities and ways of doing things.

Imagining, as discussed in Chapter 1, is part of a process of putting oneself into as yet unknown situations and considering actions and possible consequences. This might mean, when first entering into the nursing programme or a new work environment, working from a position of personal experience and imagining how to respond within some of the situations discussed in class but not as yet experienced. 'Imaging' is a way of thinking about and questioning possibilities as part of development (Parse, 2004). Reflective imagining goes further by integrating the personal with the professional, identifying the required, and possibly ideal, response and what your likely response would be by using self-knowledge, and then thinking about what and how you could develop. This is clarified through reading Marc's biographical account in the case study below.

Case study: Marc's biographical account

Marc is French by birth but has been brought up in Britain since he was seven years old because his mother's second marriage was to a British man. He is single and volunteers for a charity helpline in his spare time.

Marc is at the end of his nursing programme. As he prepares for registration he is thinking about a recent placement where he found he was able to integrate his personal and professional knowledge in a meaningful way. He was working with the district nurses and visited a young man who had been in a road traffic accident in which he lost his girlfriend, his leg and subsequently his job. After surgery and coming home, the wound had broken down and was now taking a long time to heal. Coincidentally the patient was also French, although he spoke reasonable English. On the district nursing visits to change the dressing, Marc had noticed that the patient was becoming increasingly withdrawn.

Marc tried to imagine what it must be like to lose so much so suddenly. He thought that anxiety and depression were most likely to follow but was uncertain how to approach this. He knew he had good communication skills from his charity helpline activity, but he was not a trained counsellor. He also knew that he could communicate in the patient's native language, which helped. He started by checking whether his understanding of how the patient was feeling was correct. He did not, however, have enough mental health knowledge to proceed further and suggested to his practice supervisor that a referral might be helpful.

Marc reflected on how often mental health and general nursing issues overlapped. He considered that it would be good development, both professionally and personally, to undertake a counselling course. This experience had helped him to recognise that, by integrating his personal and professional knowledge, he had been able to reach the patient in a more personal way. With *reflexivity*, the experience had also shown him where he could develop further.

Marc's biographical account illustrates how reflective imagining begins when we are uncertain of what to do. Uncertainties with unknown situations can be disturbing. Jarvis (2007, p11) calls this *disharmony*. Although this might sound undesirable, actually, uncertainty is an absolutely normal part of critical thinking and, in fact, it is what makes us question whether we can deal with a situation and whether to ask for help. In other words, it is how we risk assess situations and set boundaries as to what we can and cannot do. This prompts the imagining referred to above. Connecting with others, reflecting and imagining are all part of critical thinking. Integrated thinking means acknowledging that all experience can be useful to inform activity and, equally, different activities help to inform integrated thinking. However, thinking, as identified in Marc's account, can also create uncertainty and anxiety where gaps in knowledge are perceived. Reflection and imagining perceive such gaps, and this can stimulate uncertainty and even anxiety. As adults, and as professionals, situations of uncertainty stimulate us to seek out solutions. These experiences can be drawn together through processes of self-reflections and reflecting and imagining with others in order to expand solutions. These processes are illustrated in Figure 3.1 to represent how learning that integrates personal experience with professional experience might occur.

Integration becomes possible only when the processes of disequilibrium and seeking further information have occurred, including consulting others. The reflective practitioner incorporates imagination to support new directions that take account of feedback. When all are completed, integrative thinking draws the parts together.

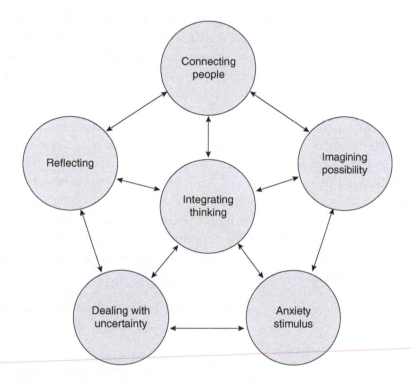

Figure 3.1 Integration of personal and professional experience
Source: Howatson-Jones (2010).

Integrative thinking uses meanings and symbolism. The first consideration is how we give meaning to a situation and communicate this to others. If our meaning is rejected by others, we may conform to their meaning as observed from their behaviour. Marc, in his account, checks his interpretation of how the patient is feeling with the patient. When meaning is discussed, others' views may be taken into consideration and used to help translate concepts. Marc can identify that the patient's feelings potentially translate into a mental health issue that needs addressing. Nevertheless, where others' interpretations become the accepted meaning, this too may become fixed and conform to behavioural norms, for example, by viewing mental health and general nursing as something entirely separate. In this instance, Marc incorporates compassion, communication and courage, three of the 6 Cs: compassion by recognising the patient's pain and possible feelings of guilt, communication by realising the importance of the patient being able to talk and share his feelings, and him possibly needing to do so in his own language, and courage by engaging in deeper interaction with the patient without knowing what his response would be or whether Marc would be able to deal with it, plus courage to decide to communicate in a language his colleague did not understand and taking the risk that the district nurse would feel excluded. Through his actions, Marc is addressing a number of important items in the section *Prioritise people* of the NMC's Code (NMC, 2018b). By paying attention to the patient's wellbeing and loss, and negotiating referral to mental health services, Marc was addressing *Prioritise people* (items 3.1, 3.3, 3.4, 4.1 and 5.4) of the NMC's Code (NMC, 2018b). Marc's actions may appear obvious, but awareness of the actual situation prompts action from the nurse. By placing the patient and his welfare centrally, applying the 6 Cs and being aware of personal strengths and limitations, the nurse can make the appropriate decisions and meet the standards of their profession.

How anxiety is managed determines whether reflective imagination is restrained by conforming behaviours or enabled by ideas continuing to develop and reach out to the unknown, while considering reflexively how the self is changing. Anxiety is the stimulant for thinking of alternatives and experimenting with change, but needs to be accompanied by self-awareness of overcoming obstacles to support positive progress. For example, Marc's confidence has increased because his practice supervisor has taken his concern seriously. These points are illustrated in a schema in Figure 3.2. The influence of anxiety is shown at the crossing points marked with an X and the arrows represent potential direction.

Review your own meaning making and development of ideas by completing Activity 3.5.

Activity 3.5   Critical thinking

- Looking back on your own life, identify a situation where you were anxious and uncertain of how to proceed, or where you were moving into a new beginning. You might consider when you were starting your nursing programme, your first day on a new placement or moving into your first qualified role after completing the programme.
- Reflect on how you made meaning of the situation. By using the schema in Figure 3.2, can you see where you might have been conforming to behavioural norms or, alternatively, where meaning is coming from developing ideas and reflexive awareness?

There is an outline answer to this activity at the end of the chapter.

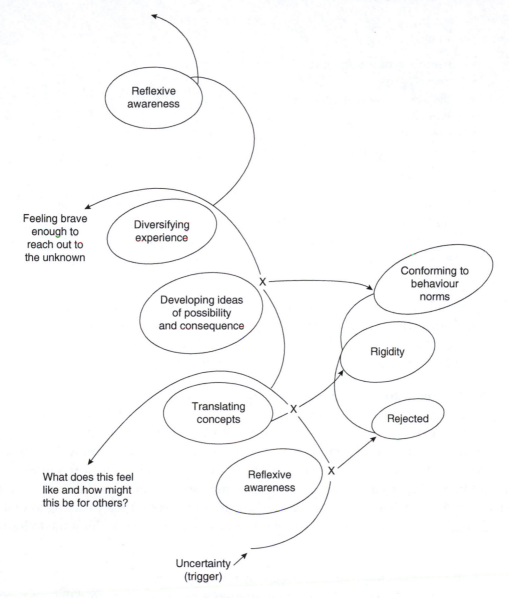

Figure 3.2 Schema of reflective imagination
Source: Howatson-Jones (2010).

Activity 3.6   Reflection

Compile a written account of your life story so far. This might include aspects such as:

- where you were born;
- family, siblings, parents, extended family;

(Continued)

(Continued)

- friends growing up and friends later on in life;
- growing up;
- significant events;
- school;
- first job;
- choice of career;
- interests.

As this activity relates to your own experience, there is no outline answer at the end of the chapter.

Having identified a few experiences from your own life and how you developed meaning, and following on from what you have learned so far about autobiographical reflection and integrating personal and professional experiences, we now proceed to a life story exercise that helps you to prepare your autobiography.

It sometimes helps to write your autobiography in the chronological order in which things happened. You may not remember everything at once, so feel free to go back to your life story and add things you may remember later. You might find it helpful to select a personal photograph or a picture from a magazine that you feel symbolises how you view the world, and then discuss the item by describing why it is important to you and how it represents your story. Illustrate the aspects you have chosen to include with examples. In talking about specific events, try to focus on their meaning as well as their factual content. When you have completed the account, think about the following questions:

- How did constructing your autobiography make you feel?
- Whose voices appear in the construction? For example, you may find that an aspect that you feel strongly about comes directly from a parent. Is this then your voice, or that of your mother, father, etc.? Or perhaps you realise that you have developed a very different idea to what you were brought up to believe. How does this realisation make you feel?
- How do you regulate emotion?
- Did you have any concerns and, if so, what were these?
- Are there elements you wish to change and, if so, why?
- What might this process tell you about working with clients/patients?

This exercise aims to help you to develop self-awareness of your values and developing professional values. For example, think about how you are developing the 6 Cs in your way of being. Having asked you to compile your autobiography, we now proceed to consider how you might examine and reflect upon its content to develop your learning.

How to examine and reflect upon autobiography

You may have taken some time to decide what to put into your autobiography. Such decisions are likely to be influenced by what the purpose is in writing it; although the exercise in this book requests you to write your autobiography, please try to remember that you are doing it for yourself, so consider what your purpose is for undertaking this activity. Your writing may also be affected by who the potential readers are and what range of experiences you have had to choose from. All these aspects are analytical points of interest when starting to examine your autobiography.

How the autobiography is structured can convey a sense of how you have been shaped by the events you have experienced and, at the same time, may also be a process of repair and change where experiences have been difficult or painful (Fischer-Rosenthal, 2000). Examination of your autobiography is a tool for developing self-awareness and reflecting upon it is a way of being able to actively influence future direction and initiate change.

It does take considerable time, effort and emotional fortitude to properly examine and reflect on your autobiography. This starts from the time of assembling it and continues through to its completion and afterwards. This process is part of a life-long activity and is, consequently, ongoing. Understanding what you need to learn, and accessing sources to achieve this, is an essential part of life-long learning. It is recommended that you return to your autobiography from time to time to understand and be aware of your development. Questions of context, feelings and knowledge base are important features in all types of reflection. However, when questioning autobiography these questions are inadequate on their own to gain sufficiently meaningful answers to what personal life brings to the situation, personal development and professional development. What is needed is also to focus on the connections between experiences past, present and future, and to examine ways in which thinking has changed or is changing, and what your personal responses to this are. Other important aspects to consider include the regulation of emotion in terms of how it is shown, by examining different 'voices' and emerging themes (Horsdal, 2012). This enables you to look at what is being internalised and how this occurs. This might seem to be quite a 'heavy' activity to undertake, but this level of reflection does help us become resilient and able to deal with the issues and challenges that we face along the way. In the *Promote professionalism and trust* section of the NMC's Code (2018b) statements address the importance of being aware of how your behaviour can impact on others (item 20.3) and the importance of maintaining an optimal level of health (item 20.9). These items resonate with Jen's story where stress and disappointment could impact on how she approaches her learning and patient care. We are all faced with challenging situations throughout our lives, but we need to build resilience in order to manage ourselves appropriately; this type of reflection allows us to build this resilience and is part of being a professional.

Scenario 3.3, Jen's biographical account, is provided to help illustrate some significant features that may be relevant to past, present and future learning and associated emotional aspects. You are asked to identify some of these features after reading the scenario.

Scenario 3.3: Jen's biographical account

Jen is in the second semester of the first year of her nursing programme after completing her A-levels. Having grown up in a town in quite a rural part of the country, she also enjoys the hustle and bustle of living in a city. She particularly enjoys the freedom of living away from home, but finds the more independent mode of study, when compared with school, challenging.

Jen grew up in a close-knit family and is the middle child of three. Her family has lived in the same place for as long as Jen can remember, and she has always been very close to her maternal grandmother who lives close to her parents. Visiting her paternal grandparents was an annual holiday treat because they lived some hours away at the coast.

Jen had always wanted to be a nurse because she saw herself being able to 'do good' and 'care for other people'. Jen's parents were supportive and encouraged her to go into nursing because of the job security that the education could provide, and they considered it a 'noble profession'. They were, however, somewhat apprehensive of their daughter moving 'so far away' and being the first in the family to go to university. Finance was another point of concern, but, as Jen had obtained very good A-levels, they felt that they did not want to stand in their daughter's way.

Jen has recently received her first assignment mark of a borderline pass and is finding her first assessed placement particularly challenging. This has left her feeling quite despondent and doubting her capabilities. She really wants to return home to be with her parents and grandmother, but knows that she cannot miss any of the placement time and she needs to be mindful of finances because she's used up too much money already on socialising with her new friends.

Activity 3.7   Identifying

* What are the significant features within this biographical account and why?

There is an outline answer to this question at the end of the chapter.

Having read Jen's biographical account and answered the question at the end, you will be able to see that examining and reflecting are not the same. Examining your autobiography means collating events and looking for particular features. It also means paying attention to the factual content. This might include questions such as the following:

- What is the timeline of events? Identifying the timeline gives clues to the different stages of your life and how these might relate to external events.
- What decisions were made? Decision-making can provide information about how you were thinking at the time.
- How is identity visible? Is there a difference between role and identity? Tracing the thread of an identity helps to raise awareness of changes and the circumstances that affect this. Do different roles call for different identities? What would this mean for you?
- Where is learning evident? Identifying learning helps to develop personal knowledge. Again, does this knowledge help you develop an identity or a particular role?

Examining your autobiography also requires you to ask more contemplative questions about the relationships between people and the construction of the story. For example, what underlie the direction and focus of the construction of your story and its inclusions? This helps in reflecting on more hidden meaning.

It is by reflecting on your autobiographical account that sense can be made from it in distinguishing between then and now, and how meaning is constantly evolving in the light of new knowledge, the connections made, strategies identified and learning taken forward. Equally, reflecting on the features within it also starts to reveal changes in your role and your identity as you develop. For example, think of your identity and role as a child and then as an adult. Although your role as a child or sibling has remained unchanged within the family, your identity has developed and, as a result, your perception of the role has altered. Your changed perception has changed the dynamics within the family structure and, through your change, you have 'demanded' that others within the family view you differently. These changes can clearly be seen during puberty. Such development can be called a process of 'becoming'. Similarly, as the novice professional grows in skill and knowledge of what it is to be a professional (identity) (Maich et al., 2000), so the perceptions of the role change and develop. Initially reflecting on the new role might include the following questions:

- Which elements from your personal history give this event significance? Look back across your life experience and review what is active. Taking note of the experiences is one way to start making the connections from which new insights emerge.
- What meaning does this have? Making sense of new insights requires defining what we mean.
- What did the environment or context contribute to this meaning? Contexts encompass objects, people, cultures and society, all of which influence behaviour and the meaning we give things.

- How do I feel about this now? Reviewing how feelings change helps to acknowledge and make sense of emotional learning and the associated development of your thinking.
- How is my identity changing? Reviewing a changing identity helps to develop self-awareness and reflexivity in how events are shaping you as a person and as a professional.
- Do you respond differently if you are expected to do something beyond your competence as a professional or if you are confronted by inappropriate behaviour? Reviewing where your boundaries lie and how you establish and maintain your boundaries is an important element of professional development.
- Are my values changing/changed? Reviewing changes in values can provide clues about societal or cultural influences that are instrumental in shaping you as a professional.

However, contemplative reflection also requires asking broader questions about the role we take in shaping our world and the role of the world in shaping us. For example, a person who has come from another country, or perhaps another region, will have an identity that is rooted in the cultural values of that place. The starting point is to reflect on what these might be in the first instance, in order to be able to identify a change and where that then stems from – whether from the person or perhaps a necessity to conform. An example you may want to reflect on would be the choices an individual may need to make in accepting and coming out in terms of sexual orientation or gender identity.

Now use these suggestions about examining and reflecting on your autobiography to complete Activity 3.8.

Activity 3.8   Critical thinking

Examine and reflect on your own autobiography, which you compiled earlier, using the suggestions above and the following questions:

- What does your autobiography contribute to your learning to be a professional?
- What potential alternative strategies does your autobiography contribute to your learning and decision-making?
- What conclusions have you reached from this exercise?
- What new insights have you developed and why?

There is an outline answer to this activity at the end of the chapter.

Having asked you to examine and reflect on your own autobiography, we now move on to consider how this relates to the perception of societal issues.

Identifying subjective perception of societal issues

Developing an autobiography can help to illustrate issues that are/were present in society at that time, and how they actually affect individuals through having a lived experience of the issues. This is one way in which an autobiography raises awareness of social processes (West, 2001). In healthcare, professionals need to be conscious of the uniqueness of each patient and the patient's lived experience of the condition and the services they have accessed, but at the same time remain aware of how individual patient health experiences contribute to a wider understanding of health issues, for example, an experience of unemployment that you have had might reveal how welfare is organised, and thought of, within societal structures. Such experiences may even change your previously held views and social values, because of the power of the message imparted through your subjective experience, which may have far-reaching and life-long effects. This can create a lens through which social issues and others' experiences can be perceived.

Critically reflecting on subjective experience is a way to (a) acknowledge its value in developing understanding and (b) reveal how personal views might have become shaped by others and become entrenched as norms. What is perceived as normal and helpful through childhood experiences may be viewed very differently when looking back more critically from adult experience (Brookfield, 2005). Such critical reflection looks back and examines issues of power surrounding events and the learning taken from them. The following case study of subjective perception of societal issues provides an illustration of such a process.

Case study: Identifying subjective perception of societal issues

Kelly is in the third year of her nursing programme. In this year the focus of the modules she is undertaking is on developing skills in leadership and managing care, and on making the transition into practice. Kelly has had a recent placement within a surgical ward. She managed the care of a number of women. One in particular, Jane, has troubled her and she is trying to critically reflect on the situation, which has led her to question her own values and those of society.

Jane was admitted, by Kelly, for an excision breast biopsy of a suspected breast cancer. Jane also had learning disabilities and so attended with her carer. Kelly is puzzled by this. She has a brother with learning disabilities and he has always lived with the family and gone to a mainstream school. Kelly starts to admit Jane by talking to her directly, but the carer intervenes, answering on her behalf. Kelly completes Jane's admission

(Continued)

(Continued)

and starts to prepare her for the procedure. Clearly Jane is frightened and confused by what is happening, so Kelly takes some time to sit with her and explain what she is doing. She uses her drawing skills to show Jane what she means when it is apparent that Jane does not understand, and she does the same when the surgeon and anaesthetist come to see her. Kelly accompanies Jane to theatre and collects her as well to ensure that she sees a familiar face.

When reflecting on this incident, there are a number of issues that come to the fore for Kelly. She sees the person, not the deficit. She has also noticed the limited response of the surgeon and anaesthetist when faced by Jane's incomprehension. She wonders whether the voice of the learning-disabled service user is heard by those aiming to care for her. When reflecting on her own experience, Kelly realises that her own values and beliefs of seeing the person rather than a deficit are based on her experiences with her brother. She had assumed that these values are more mainstream because her brother's school friends accept him as he is.

Having seen the difficulty that there is within certain institutions, such as the hospital, she questions whether these difficulties also stem from a society that is less comfortable with difference and does not, therefore, offer appropriate provision according to person-centred need, but rather according to deficit. Kelly looks at why her values are different. She has grown up with her brother and knows him and his ways. Would she find his outbursts frightening if she did not know him? She wonders how much of this is related to control. Is a deficit model a kind of control? Kelly realises that control comes in many forms, not least in building relationships.

In this case study Kelly has identified disharmony between her taken-for-granted values and those she is experiencing in her student practitioner role. This has led her to reflect on why societal values might differ from hers and to question her assumptions. From such a position Kelly can advocate more effectively for her patient by entering into the societal debate more knowledgeably. You are advised to find items from the NMC's Code (2018b) that relate to Kelly's situation, for example, in the sections *Prioritise people* (items 1.1, 1.3, 1.5, 2.1–2.4, 2.6 and 3.4) and *Promote professionalism* (items 20.5 and 20.7). Please complete Activity 3.9 to identify some of your own values and assumptions.

Activity 3.9   Critical thinking

Can you think of experiences in your own life that helped to develop your understanding of some social issues? Reflect on these by looking at the following questions. To help you with this activity, you may want to consider the 'protected characteristics' (Equality Act 2010) as a starting point.

- What were the assumptions surrounding the situation?
- What values were active in the situation?
- What did you learn about the social issue?
- Has anything changed as a result of this learning?

There is an outline answer to this activity at the end of the chapter.

Having identified your own assumptions and values through the activity and by reflecting on the learning you have achieved in the situations you reflected on, you may potentially be able to be a more effective advocate for your patient in similar circumstances.

Chapter summary

This chapter has explained the ways in which autobiography can contribute to learning as a professional. By offering a number of suggestions of how to compile, examine and reflect on a personal biography, the chapter provided the starting and developing healthcare professional with the possibility of integrating personal and professional experiences into something meaningful to their learning. In this way it becomes possible to better understand personal learning needs and objectives and developing professional values, and to recognise a developing identity.

Activities and scenarios: Brief outline answers

Activity 3.1 Callum's biographical account of school (Scenario 3.2, page 50)

The learning Callum possibly has taken forward is:

- formal learning can be painful and confusing;
- it is difficult to trust and feel comfortable with peers;
- it is important to be helpful and caring in order to be accepted by others.

Activity 3.2 Reflection on Callum's biographical account of school (Scenario 3.2, page 52)

The meaning that Callum is likely to have attached is the following:

- Learning at school was a struggle.
- He can inspire others.
- He can trust people to support him.
- Asking for help can be difficult.

- It is difficult to trust that others will provide support.
- Asking for support can be a good thing.

Some creative strategies that Callum could employ might be:

- to focus on trying to articulate the subjects he needs to learn, as if he were motivating a rugby team;
- to realise that everyone has their strengths and role to play within a group;
- to try to break down the task he needs to learn into smaller parts and understand what support he needs to be successful;
- to work with others as study partners;
- to use his sense of tactics to plan his learning and manage his time;
- to talk things over with lecturers and practice supervisors;
- to be open and honest with colleagues, lecturers and practice supervisors.

Activity 3.3 Critical thinking (page 53)

Your answer might have related to the following key points:

- recognising important relationships;
- acknowledging emotional blocks and drivers in learning;
- developing understanding of strengths and areas of development;
- developing self-knowledge.

Activity 3.5 Critical thinking (page 58)

When thinking about first starting the nurse preparation programme or moving into practice, you might have included:

- needing to identify what was expected by your practice supervisor and practice colleagues or, perhaps, by the regulatory body;
- professional behaviours;
- knowledge base.

When considering integrating thinking, you might have included:

- fitting into the team and learning what it means to be a healthcare professional;
- working interprofessionally to gain a wider perspective;
- reflecting on reasons for anxiety and uncertainty and addressing knowledge gaps;
- integrating reflective and imaginative ideas.

Activity 3.7 Identifying significant features in Jen's autobiographical account (page 62)

This scenario includes the following features, which provide a good starting point for further examination and reflection on what is brought to the nursing course and how this is progressing:

- moving from a town to a new city;
- changing study experiences;
- enjoying social processes;
- loss of parental and family support networks;
- teaching and leadership skills;
- being responsible and accountable for actions and choices;
- self-reliance.

Activity 3.8 Critical thinking (page 64)

You might have addressed this activity by considering events about difficulty, how the past has been overcome, and how you are taking something forward into the future in a more positive way. Or you might have used a cautionary tale of how not to proceed, or a moral story of the right thing to do. Reflection may have included looking at emotional as well as cognitive learning, and how your identity is developing.

Activity 3.9 Critical thinking (pages 66–7)

Answers to the activity are likely to have centred around:

- values such as dignity and respect, person-centredness, compassion and holistic care;
- assumptions;
- societal views;
- learning.

Further reading

Dominice, P (2000) *Learning from Ourselves*. San Francisco, CA: Jossey-Bass.

This book identifies how preparing an educational biography can help with understanding processes of learning.

Formenti, L, West, L and Horsdal, M (eds) (2014) *Embodied Narratives: Connecting stories, bodies, cultures and ecologies*. Odense: University of Southern Denmark Press.

This book focuses on issues about the body and emotions and their relationship to thinking, areas that are often neglected in adult learning. It usefully sets parts within a whole by considering identity, culture, theories, imagination and ideas about professionalism.

Horsdal, M (2012) *Telling Lives: Exploring dimensions of narratives*. London: Routledge.

This book identifies the relevance and importance of how we construct our biographies to tell others who we are and why we respond in certain ways.

Chapter 4 Reflective models and frameworks

NMC Standards of Proficiency for Registered Nurses

This chapter will address the following platforms and proficiencies:

Platform 1: Being an accountable professional

1.17 Take responsibility for continuous self-reflection, seeking and responding to support and feedback to develop their professional knowledge and skills.

Platform 5: Leading and managing nursing care and working in teams

5.10 Contribute to supervision and team reflection activities to promote improvements in practice and services.

Platform 6: Improving safety and quality of care

6.12 Understand the role of registered nurses and other health and care professionals at different levels of experience and seniority when managing and prioritising actions and care in the event of a major incident.

Chapter aims

After reading this chapter you will be able to:

- identify different models and frameworks of reflection;
- consider strengths and limitations of different models and frameworks;
- choose an appropriate model or framework for your reflection.

Introduction

Scenario 4.1: Jane's use of empathy

Jane was working in an outpatient department in the second year of her nursing programme. She had spent some time talking to a young woman – Sarah – in the waiting area who looked emotional, tense and nervous. Sarah, who was in her early 30s, was waiting to see the consultant about a lump in her left breast. Jane's practice supervisor James asked Sarah if she would mind Jane sitting in on her consultation. Sarah agreed, becoming quite tearful.

The consultant examined Sarah and asked her what she thought the lump could be. Jane said she was concerned that she might have breast cancer because the lump had been there now for some time and her grandmother had died from metastasised breast cancer, at which point Sarah began to cry in earnest. The consultant listened to Sarah's concerns and said that, although this was one possibility, there were other causes for a breast lump and he wanted to complete some tests first. He explained the tests to Sarah. However, the consultant realised that Sarah did not appear to be absorbing or processing all this information, and he asked Jane to get Sarah some refreshment and some explanatory leaflets while he saw the next patient. Jane sat with Sarah while she tried to read some of the leaflets, and offered to help Sarah write down any questions she may have. The consultant then saw Sarah again to answer her questions. Jane was a little taken aback by this second consultation in what seemed to be a busy clinic. At the end of the day she discussed her impressions with James. Jane said she had not seen a doctor work in this way on other placements – unhurried and interested even though he had a long list of people to see. James asked Jane to reflect on the differences she had noticed in the way this consultant worked and what the potential outcomes might be for the patients, the staff and the organisation.

That evening Jane spent some time reflecting on her day. She began by thinking about how she had seen other healthcare professionals interact with patients and what differences she had noticed with this consultant. She noted that the consultant completely focused on Sarah and was not trying to write, or look at the computer or notes, at the same time. She also noted that he had attentively listened to Jane's concerns about the lump and had given her time to absorb his explanation and ask further questions. Jane thought this was a good idea because she remembered her first experience of having a cervical smear test, not really understanding the results, and feeling frustrated that no one would really listen to her or explain what they were doing. Jane wondered whether the consultant had perhaps experienced being a service user himself or had experienced similar situations with family members that might explain his actions.

(Continued)

(Continued)

Jane continued to ponder on these thoughts for a while. She considered that the outcome for Sarah would be feeling that her concerns had been listened to. Jane thought that staff would find the consultant as approachable as she had, and that the organisation would benefit through such a collegiate, interprofessional atmosphere contributing to a positive workplace culture. Jane considered what she was taking forward from reflecting on this experience. It was the realisation of how important attentive listening is to good patient care. She spoke about this with James the next day when they discussed her reflection. James agreed and added that focusing on the positives of the situation would enable her to use this approach within her practice. The next day Jane observed an elderly woman – Mrs Scott – in the waiting room looking anxiously at the clock while she waited for her dermatology appointment. She tentatively approached the service user and began a conversation. Jane tried to focus on listening attentively to Mrs Scott, trying not to look too pointedly at the skin discolorations on her hands, arm and neck. Jane was aware of thinking that they looked very itchy and thought of how embarrassed she would be if she had a condition that was so visible to others. One of the first things that Mrs Scott said was that her husband had dementia and that she was his primary carer. She was anxious to get back home. Jane was able to add this information to the consultation, which had, until then, focused purely on physical results, enabling the consideration of stress as a potential underlying cause of Mrs Scott's symptoms.

Activity 4.1   Reflection

To get into the 'reflective zone', imagine yourself in Jane's position or in an actual situation that you have experienced. Briefly write this down so that you have a set scenario to work from. Once you have a clear idea of the situation in your mind, jot down some answers to the following questions:

- What goes through your mind when you are with someone of a similar age who is distressed about their situation? Then move on to how do you feel when you are in this situation. Are your thoughts and emotions similar or are they different? Try to think back as to how you behaved in this situation. Were you aware of being influenced by your thoughts and/ or emotions? (For example, did you find yourself becoming emotional as well? Did this, perhaps, result in you becoming a little more distant or formal? Was this, in your opinion 'professional' behaviour in this situation? Why and on what do you base this idea?)
- Do you respond in the same way with someone much older than yourself? If yes, why? If no, why not? Try to think of this in terms of how you would interpret 'patient-centred care'.

As this is a reflective exercise for yourself, there is no outline answer at the end of the chapter.

The example offered above demonstrates how situations, that arouse emotions, can stimulate thinking about them. The example will be reworked further through using *reflective cycles*, to help demonstrate different stages of a reflective process. Using models and reflective cycles can help you, especially if you are less experienced, to develop your reflection into something that enables you to really examine your learning.

This chapter introduces some of the wide range of reflective models and frameworks that you can draw from when first starting, to structure and frame your reflections. You will be encouraged to consider some of the strengths and limitations of the selected reflective frameworks, models and cycles, to help you to choose appropriately. The right questions to ask will also be highlighted through the example and case study presented.

Reflective frameworks

Donald Schön (1991) examined how professionals think about what they are doing and described these ways of thinking as reflection-in-action and reflection-on-action. When in a situation, we are constantly reworking problems and discovering consequences from this reworking, and these have implications for further adaptations. Schön (1991) identifies this as a framing process whereby, through reframing roles and perspectives of a situation, new phenomena come into view and can be worked in other ways that may bring different solutions. In the example, Jane observes a positive communication style that she recognises as contrasting with the pressured version with which she is more familiar. By recognising the benefits for the patient, the organisation and herself, and using her analysis to reframe her future communications, Jane reflects on how her attitude and communication could allow her to contribute effectively to the workplace. This is often known as reflection before action and Jane had this in mind when she tentatively approached Mrs Scott. It was quite understandable for Jane to feel a little apprehensive when approaching a service user initially. In starting a conversation with Mrs Scott, Jane would become aware of how Mrs Scott communicated with her: her intonation, non-verbal communication and choice of words. Naturally, Jane would not know which direction the interaction would take but, using the cues she received from Mrs Scott and the communication theory she had covered, Jane felt that she would have been able to respond appropriately to Mrs Scott's concerns. Reflection-in-action can, therefore, be described as a form of experimentation in problem solving that acknowledges uncertainty and looks at discovering potential answers or ways to proceed. Schön (1991, p76) describes this as having a *reflective conversation with the situation*, which is also the strength of this approach, in that it is working with the situation in real time. In other words, we are constantly interpreting and responding to cues within the situation and consequently changing its course in the process. Nevertheless, a limitation is that much of this reflection often occurs unconsciously as part of working with experience intuitively. 'Intuitively' means that articulated descriptions can never fully explain the actions taken or knowledge used, or *artistry* involved (Schön, 1991, p276). Undertaking Activity 4.2 will help you to understand these points.

Activity 4.2   Evidence-based practice and reflection

Observe someone undertaking an activity. It might be your practice supervisor in practice or a lecturer in class. If you are an experienced practitioner, it might be an advanced practitioner in their field. Consider how their activity flows and whether they seem to be aware of each process or step they are undertaking. For example, think about the following.

- When is it obvious to you that they have in some way modified their actions?
- Were there hesitations when they might have thought about what they were doing and altered direction?
- What happened when you, or somebody else, asked them a question?
- How was the answer worked out?

There is an outline answer to this activity at the end of the chapter.

The process of reflection-in-action enables adaptation of learning from experience during action. Critical analysis, which will be explored as critical reflection in more detail in Chapter 11, helps to formalise and record these processes. When completing nursing activities yourself, you may have become aware that you are not conscious of thoughts at the time, but that you are responding to what you think the situation might require. This is because, when we stop, we become more aware of what is going on in our thinking as well as acting. We also become conscious of what we have learned through the action we have undertaken, when looking back on it. Schön (1991) suggests that thinking too much about action, while undertaking it, might raise barriers to the smooth flow of the action. Although you may feel that thinking about your every move limits your activity, you might want to bear in mind that, when learning new skills or activities, it is completely normal that you need to think through each step. You will find that, as you gain experience, you will be able to think things through (reflection-in-action) at the same time as undertaking the activity. However, equally beneficial to your learning is to look back at the action. This can help the professional gain greater insight and clarity in their thought processes and the actions taken. This is called reflection-on-action. As seen in Scenario 4.1 the process of reflection-on-action highlights the learning achieved for future use and is particularly useful for the novice to undertake. Completing Activity 4.3 may help you to identify some of your own learning from reflection-on-action.

As you completed Activity 4.3 you might have become aware of aspects that were, perhaps, not obvious to you at the time of the event. Or you may have identified gaps in your knowledge. In the next section we consider how using a reflective model can help you to question some of these elements in order to develop your learning and to question the evidence base that supports what you are doing.

Activity 4.3   Critical thinking

Think of Scenario 4.1 and try to work through the questions below. After doing this, reflect on whether the type of question you have as a cue influences how you reflect and whether you identify different elements as important.

After you've done this, choose a recent patient-related situation when you worked with your practice supervisor or, if you are an experienced practitioner, think of a time when you worked with a student. Consider a patient-related problem that you dealt with together.

- What was the patient problem?
- Was the problem clear to you both at the start?
- Were there different interpretations of the problem during the situation?
- How did this become clear?
- Were you conscious of this during the situation?
- What discoveries did you make during the situation?
- How did these influence your further actions?
- How did your further actions act on the problem?
- What learning are you taking away from the situation?

There is an outline answer to this activity at the end of the chapter.

Reflective models

Reflection requires some effort and practice to maintain the necessary focus on thoughts, feelings and memories for making appropriate changes (Taylor, 2010). For example, you might find it emotionally difficult when dealing with death and dying. It could be useful to use a model because it will help you to identify key stages of your reflective learning. The structure of a model can provide you with footholds that help you to keep going when you are dealing with complex issues, in order to arrive at a resolution about how to deal with the situation. It is important to choose a model that suits your needs and that you find easy to use. Nevertheless, for reflection to be of value and to maintain progression in your life-long learning, it is important to regularly reflect on what you are doing and, on your learning. In fact, we should all strive to embed reflection as an integral part of who we are as learners and practitioners. In other words, reflection should become a way of being – second nature – rather than something that you do as an add-on or because you need to include it in an assignment.

In Chapter 1 we referred to Barksby et al. (2015), who suggest a new model of reflection for clinical practice, but we also suggested that this 'new' approach is built on earlier, seminal models. As such, it is beneficial to have some understanding of the development of reflective thinking in nursing and the following models offer several perspectives, areas on which to focus your reflection and questions you might want to ask yourself. The principles of the models are similar and they all provide a framework and cue questions to support reflective thinking, so try to be selective when choosing a model to work with because, besides personal preference, the situation and context could lend itself better to one model rather than another.

Johns (2013) has developed and refined the following model over a number of years through working with many practitioners at different stages of their development. This is an important point to realise: reflection is dynamic and the ways in which it is undertaken are constantly evolving. Therefore, any model can only ever be a guide rather than an ending in itself.

Model for Structured Reflection

The Model for Structured Reflection (MSR; Johns, 2013) identifies how you might want to examine your experience more extensively and in greater depth in order to really learn from it. The model's starting point is to create space for reflection – what Johns (2013) calls *bringing the mind home*, which means stilling the mind so it can focus. The model then encompasses a number of reflective cues, or questions, which the practitioner is asked to think about in the course of reflecting on a situation. These are presented below.

Concept summary: MSR reflective cues

- Bringing the mind home.
- Description of positive and problematic issues.
- Reflection on what occurred in terms of the following:

  o What issues are significant to pay attention to?
  o How were others feeling and why did they feel that way?
  o How was I feeling and what made me feel that way?
  o What was I trying to achieve and did I respond effectively?
  o What were the consequences of my actions on the patient, others and myself?
  o To what extent did I act for the best and in tune with my values?
  o What knowledge did or might have informed me?
  o How does this situation connect with previous experiences?
  o What assumptions govern my practice and what factors influence the way I feel, think and respond to the particular situation?

Anticipation in terms of:

- How might I reframe the situation in order to respond more effectively?
- What would be the consequences of responding differently for the patient, others and myself?
- What factors might constrain me responding in new ways?
- How do I NOW feel about this experience?

Insights in terms of:

- What insights have I gained? (framing perspectives)

(Source: Johns, 2013)

These cues encompass aesthetic, personal, ethical, empirical and reflexive aspects that are related to Carper's (1978) fundamental patterns of knowing (Johns, 1995):

- Aesthetics relates to how the person feels about, responds to and perceives the situation and those involved.
- Personal aspects explore, from the person, what was influencing them.
- Ethics encompasses how actions are related to beliefs.
- Empirics are concerned with what knowledge was used.
- Reflexivity relates to how experiences are connected and the possible alternatives and changes to doing things differently.

The following case study makes use of these cues to help illustrate how this model might be applied.

Case study: Tamara's experience of comforting

Tamara was working on a gynaecology ward and her practice supervisor had arranged for her to spend some time in the early pregnancy unit with the scanning nurse, Pip. Pip scanned a lady called Monica and found that there was no fetal heartbeat. When she informed Monica of this she was understandably very upset. Pip asked Tamara to stay with Monica while she made further arrangements.

Tamara took Monica somewhere quiet where they could talk in private. She thought that Monica would probably want to be away from prying eyes. Tamara began by saying

(Continued)

(Continued)

how sorry she was and that it was OK for Monica to express her feelings. Monica began to cry quietly. Tamara sat close to her, but not touching, because she was not sure how Monica would react to a stranger as she did not like strangers touching her. She allowed Monica to cry for a while and then asked her if she wanted anyone to be contacted. Monica said her partner was at work and she did not want to disturb him. She asked why the miscarriage had happened. Tamara explained that she was a student nurse and would get Pip. At that moment Pip came into the room to explain the next steps. She told Monica that the reasons for miscarriage are often not known, although further tests would be carried out. Both Pip and Monica thanked Tamara for being there.

Later that day Tamara's link tutor, Lynne, came to the ward. She could see that Tamara looked upset, so she took her to a quiet area to talk. Tamara told Lynne about her morning and how it had upset her. She felt that she should have done more but was not sure what she could have done. Lynne helped Tamara to reflect on the situation. They identified that Tamara had used a person-centred approach by offering Jane privacy and giving her time to express her feelings. Tamara had not imposed her own views of the situation and had sought help when asked questions that were outside her sphere of knowledge. Lynne asked Tamara what she had learned from the situation. Tamara said that the overriding thing she had learned was that we do not always have answers. She felt she could perhaps have done more in comforting Jane. Lynne and Tamara explored the options of using touch. Lynne advised Tamara to revisit communication literature. Tamara felt less upset and thought that, next time, she would talk to her practice supervisor about the situation. Nevertheless, she felt she had handled a difficult situation well.

The case study illustrates how reflection can also affirm actions as well as correct them. Using this model helps to expose how others might also be thinking and how to deal with it. This is an important point to consider in a little more depth. Often, we reflect on situations that have not gone well or where we think that there could be room for improvement. Although this is, undoubtedly, important, we should not forget that most of what we do is of good quality, achieves appropriate outcomes and receives a high score on patient satisfaction. It is, therefore, also important to reflect on things that have gone well because these situations can offer cues as to what works successfully and what our strengths are and, consequently, allows us to develop a broad range of 'tried and tested' approaches to situations. One might say that this is how we build our intuition but the strength in this would arguably be our ability to make conscious use of in-, on- or before-action reflection.

Stages of reflection

We move on now to consider another model by Atkins and Murphy (1995), which examines three main stages to reflection based on feelings, knowledge and coming to new ways of thinking.

- Stage 1: awareness of uncomfortable feelings;
- Stage 2: critical analysis of the situation;
- Stage 3: development of new perspectives on the situation.

Stage 1 of this model relates to uncomfortable feelings being the stimulus for starting to reflect on what is causing them and what can be done. Part of this will be an assessment of your knowledge base and whether this was sufficient. Atkins and Murphy (1995) make the point here that feelings need not necessarily be negative but can be more positively related to some achievement. It might be useful to qualify this point with reference to Jarvis (2007, p3) who describes such a state as 'disharmony'. This occurs when there is a break with familiar experience that alerts the person reflecting to change taking place. In other words, experiencing something for the first time can make you feel strange and uncomfortable, or perhaps you are unsure about what is expected of you or what you can or should expect from yourself.

Stage 2 relates to you examining your use of knowledge and any potential gaps there may be in your knowledge. Also, in Stage 2, you would identify how the situation made you feel and, conversely, how you may have influenced the situation through your experience or inexperience. The purpose here is to connect feelings, knowledge and information with the situation and the individual so that the person can develop new insights.

Stage 3 clarifies what these insights are by describing them as 'outcomes of reflection' and how this learning will be taken forward (Atkins and Murphy, 1995, p2).

Model of reflection from a student's perspective

Another model that you might find useful is the one developed by Stephenson and described in the chapter by Stephenson and Holm (1994) in the book by Palmer et al. (1994). This is based on students questioning their roles, feelings, actions, expectations and knowledge, as well as some of the broader surrounding issues within which their experiences may be embedded. These questions are extremely relevant to your stage of learning and are particularly helpful through asking you to relate your professional practice to the wider political and social world, which may exert influence over what is happening and what you can do.

The main questions of Stephenson's model are as shown in the box.

Concept summary: Stephenson's model of reflection (from a student's perspective)

- What was my role in the situation?
- Did I feel comfortable or uncomfortable? Why?
- What actions did I take?
- How did I and others act?
- Was it appropriate?
- How could I have improved the situation for myself, the patient, my practice supervisor?
- How can I change in future?
- Do I feel as if I have learned anything new about myself?
- Did I expect anything different to happen? What and why?
- Has it changed my way of thinking in any way?
- What knowledge from theory and research can I apply to this situation?
- What broader issues, for example political or social, arise from this situation?
- What do I think about these broader issues?

(Source: Stephenson, 1993, cited in Palmer et al., 1994)

The more experienced practitioner might want to use these questions with students as part of the teaching and assessing process to develop reflective learning together.

The final model, offered by Howatson-Jones (2010), suggests some exploratory questions that are meant to stimulate reflective thinking from a broader historical sense. These stem from personal research and are particularly relevant to reflections about working with people.

Concept summary: A biographical perspective on reflection

- What foreknowledge did I bring to the situation and what do I need to know?
- What action did I take in the situation and why?
- How might others' perceptions be framing their responses?
- What is the quality of the response and how does it make me feel and act?
- What connections are there between responses now and earlier?
- Are there contraindications? Why?

- What, from autobiography, is influencing my noticing?
- What other factors might be influencing the situation?
- What does the language used in, or about, the situation reveal?
- What dimensions does my learning take, for example, psychological, physiological, affective (behavioural), spiritual or biographical?

(Source: Howatson-Jones, 2010)

The questions offered in the Howatson-Jones (2010) model provide an excellent opportunity to reflect on how your biography can be active in what you notice and how you might reflect. In Scenario 4.1 Jane brings her foreknowledge of other doctor–patient interactions to reflect on the differences in the consultant's communication. She also thinks about possible reasons for his different attitude based on her own autobiographical experience of having been a patient herself. This is an important point to question to ensure that blind spots do not develop, because these can hinder the ability to respond in better ways. Equally, developing biographical understanding can help you to read situations in different ways and understand why the consultant's approach might work better in one area than another.

The term 'model' is sometimes used interchangeably with the term 'reflective cycle'. In essence, both offer structure to help you examine your reflective learning. Some, however, are more cyclical and are therefore referred to as reflective cycles. We proceed now to explore some reflective cycles.

Reflective cycles

Reflective cycles offer the possibility to connect what has been learned from one experience with that of another. Using a reflective cycle can help you to clarify how learning is progressing and what you need to do to support it further, and it enables you to plan further action and set objectives relating to this. There are a number of different reflective cycles that you can choose from and use. One of the most well-known reflective cycles is that of Gibbs (1988), which outlines specific steps to guide the learner through processes of description, acknowledgement of feelings, evaluation, analysis and action planning, as outlined in Figure 4.1.

The description of the situation is limited to the salient points, which are the main priorities. By acknowledging feelings, the learner can consider processes, such as how to deal with sometimes difficult emotions that may be aroused by caring work and learning. Evaluation begins to think about what the main issues are. These can then be analysed in greater detail by considering what knowledge is available, or might need to be developed, what other choices might have been accessible in the situation and the possible consequences if one of those choices had been chosen instead. From this analysis follows consideration of changes to thinking about this type of situation, and how maybe to proceed the next time. From here, further action is then planned. The important aspects of this cycle are that analysis should result in some kind of action planning to take learning forward.

Now apply Gibbs' reflective cycle to Scenario 4.1 at the start of the chapter by completing Activity 4.3.

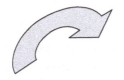
Focus – description of the issue

Action plan to take forward

Feelings produced

Evaluation of change in feelings and knowledge

Initial evaluation

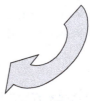

Analysis of the situation, the knowledge used and possible alternatives

Figure 4.1   Adapted from Gibbs' (1988) reflective cycle

Activity 4.4   Reflective cycle: reflection

- Using the key stages of Gibbs' (1988) reflective cycle, identify which parts of Scenario 4.1 fit with these key stages. It might help to write these out on a separate piece of paper.
- Now underline the actual words within the parts of the example that represent the action points of the key stages of the reflective cycle under which you have placed them.

There is an outline answer to this activity at the end of the chapter.

From applying Gibbs' (1988) reflective cycle to Scenario 4.1, you might have identified that Jane needed to learn more about attentive listening to develop her own communication skills. A developed cycle based on Gibbs can be found in the Davis model, which includes an additional stage of considering the evidence base for change (Davis et al., 2011). You are directed to the book *Learning Skills for Nursing Students* (Davis et al., 2011), also in this series, to learn more. We proceed now to look at a different reflective cycle.

Driscoll's (2007, p44) reflective cycle has its roots in experiential learning and views reflection as a process of interrogating:

* What?
* So what?
* Now what?

These three questions encompass the need to be clear in the interpretation, interrogation and presentation of learning through reflection. The 'what?' refers to being able to describe the situation in words. This requires some mental ordering of events and helps to start the reflective process. In Scenario 4.1 Jane has started to build a therapeutic relationship with Sarah in the waiting room and then attends her consultation with her permission. She was surprised by the consultant's communication approach because it was different to what she had previously experienced. The 'so what?' involves beginning to analyse important aspects of the experience from which new discoveries may appear. When Jane starts to analyse what is important in this situation, she becomes aware that it is the quality of attentive listening, which the consultant demonstrated, that is different to other healthcare professional/patient interactions of which she has been part. The 'now what?' proposes new actions based on these discoveries, which may be reworked in multiple different situations. Jane realises that, in the past, she has not always been really attending to what patients are saying to her and that this is a skill she needs to practise and use within her communication in the future. Driscoll's (2007) cycle is simple, but effective. It is easy to remember, and these questions can easily be asked as part of most conversations within the classroom or practice and, therefore, can multiply the opportunities for reflection.

As suggested earlier, you may have noticed some similarities for the various frameworks, models and cycles of reflection. The next cycle acknowledges this point and is founded on the main principles we have looked at so far.

Jasper (2003, p2) suggests that most cycles of reflection are founded on the principles of experience–reflection–action (ERA). The reflective cycle starts with some kind of experience or situation in which you are, or have been, involved. Experience may be something recent or something that you have developed. Reflection relates to reviewing and looking at the familiar, as well as the unfamiliar, with fresh eyes in order to consider what resources are available to you, who is, or needs to be, involved and what other strategies are available to you. Action refers to the implementation of learning and new strategies. These cycles of reflection may spiral from one to another over a period of time (Jasper, 2003), forming part of a process of becoming as the person develops themselves and their knowledge (Johns, 2013). In other words, by connecting learning from different reflective episodes, you will be in a better position to get a clearer view of how you are developing your knowledge of yourself, your profession, your environment and your culture, and of other people, as well as the theoretical knowledge that underpins this. Reflection is about being able to connect experience with what you do.

Having looked at a number of different *reflective frameworks*, models and cycles, please complete Activity 4.4 in order to clarify your understanding of them.

Activity 4.5   Critical thinking

- What are the main commonalities and differences for the various frameworks, models and cycles?
- Which of them appear easier to use and why?
- Which of them appear harder to use and why?
- Are there different types of situations that the different frameworks, models and cycles are suited to? If so, why?
- What do you see as the strengths and limitations of each of the frameworks, models and cycles?

There is an outline answer to this activity at the end of the chapter.

Chapter summary

This chapter has introduced and explored several different reflective frameworks, models and cycles that you can choose from when starting or continuing to reflect.

Through Scenario 4.2, the case study and activities provided you have been given the opportunity to apply a variety of reflective formats. These are not an end in themselves, but offer you a starting point from which to develop your own reflective journey. Nevertheless, they assist with structuring what might sometimes be painful and difficult to admit to yourself, as well as help you to identify how to replicate and multiply successes. When time is short, the discipline of a reflective framework can help to keep you on track. How to create space for such reflection is explored in greater depth in the next chapter.

Activities: Brief outline answers

Activity 4.2 Evidence-based practice and reflection (page 74)

You might have observed that your practice supervisor, teacher or advanced practitioner could talk around the subject effortlessly while undertaking the tasks of practice or teaching. You might, for example, have noted your practice supervisor adjusting a wound dressing technique in response to the patient wincing, all the while telling them what the wound dressing was for and how the wound healing was progressing. Similarly, you might have been in a clinical science class and observed the lecturer responding to some people's confusion by asking class members to take on the role of oxygen and sit in a haemoglobin 'car' made up of four chairs that could take four passengers. You might have observed the advanced practitioner skilfully completing an examination while teaching the patient and you. There might have been a fleeting hesitation while the practice supervisor, teacher or advanced practitioner took in the cues they received from the patient/class, but the alteration in what they did next would have been imperceptible. However, if the patient asks a question of the practice supervisor or a student asks the lecturer, there is a more perceptible pause to think of the answer to give. The answer is likely to have involved some dialogue to check whether it met the expectation of the questioner and that they also understood the answer.

Activity 4.3 Critical thinking (page 75)

You might have considered a patient problem relating to a developing pressure sore. You and your practice supervisor or your student may have noted a change in skin colour and appearance. There may have been a difference in interpretation of the severity of the problem due to difference in knowledge. You may not have realised this until comparing the scores you took, and you might have discovered that, when using some scoring systems, it is easy to overestimate risk. You might have been surprised by the degree of subjectivity still involved. If you are an experienced practitioner, you might have considered your accountability should the patient develop a pressure sore. You might have been more careful to regularly assess the risk using the same tool each time to monitor changes. You may have learned that assessment tools are only as good as the knowledge and observation of the person using them. In your reflection try to relate your scenario to the NMC's Code (NMC, 2018b), for example, *Practise effectively* (items 10.2 and 10.3) and *Preserve safety* (items 13.1 and 13.2).

As suggested in Scenario 4.1, in Activity 4.1 and again in this activity, much of our learning occurs through experience. This is often an unconscious process, which, as a professional engaged in life-long learning, we need to make more of a conscious process. This is where the activities of reflection-in-action and reflection-on-action become very important. This process can, however, become quite difficult to unpick and you might find it interesting to read Patricia Benner's (1984) influential work in which she discusses the process 'from novice to expert' in terms of learning. It is good to be mindful that one of Benner's key premises is that, as we develop, we tend to 'read' situations in context rather than in isolation. It may then be beneficial to you, when discussing something you have seen a colleague (this could be your practice supervisor, your student or another healthcare professional) do, to try to reduce the activity into smaller stages, in order to discuss the underlying decision-making associated with each step and how this information informed their next step.

Activity 4.4 Reflective cycle using Scenario 4.1 (page 82)

Description

Jane was working in an outpatient department in the second year of her nurse preparation programme. The consultant examined Sarah and listened to her concerns and then explained further processes. He allowed Sarah time to develop further questions.

Feelings

Jane was surprised by the empathetic communication style used by the consultant.

Evaluation

Jane noted that the consultant had attended to what Sarah was saying and how Sarah was processing the information he gave her. Jane wondered why the consultant behaved so differently to her previous experience of such consultations.

Analysis

Looking back Jane wondered whether the consultant had himself been a patient at some time and been frustrated at the way people communicated with him. Or perhaps a family member or friend had been the patient and he had tried to support them. She considered how different the consultant had been in the way he had attended to what Sarah was saying, and to her body language revealing she was feeling overwhelmed, and how the consultant had allowed Sarah time to absorb what he was being told and gain the answers to her questions. Jane thought about the impact the consultant's communication style had on making Sarah feel listened to, and the positive working atmosphere of the team. She identified that what she was seeing was an effective working culture in action. In reflecting on this scenario, it is recommended that you refer to the NMC's Code (NMC, 2018b), for example, *Prioritise people* (items 1.1, 1.5 and 2.6) and *Practise effectively* (items 8.3 and 8.6).

Evaluation of change

Jane thought about how she could develop her own attentive listening to enhance her practice.

Action planning

Jane would read more about communication, particularly in relation to attentive listening. Jane would continue to reflect on her experiences and keep a reflective log of her progress to discuss with her practice supervisor.

Activity 4.5: Critical thinking (page 84)

- You are likely to have identified that the areas of commonality between the different reflective formats include evaluation, analysis and action. Areas of difference might, for you, be in the depth of reflection demanded by the models compared with the easier application of the reflective cycles. The biographical model is also different in asking you to identify what is active in your noticing.
- You may have found reflection-in-action particularly relevant to starting to develop your practice skills, whereas reflection-on-action may have helped you to embed them. The reflective cycles might have helped you to structure reflection within assignments and when talking about practice. The models of reflection might have helped you to examine your learning in more detail through reflective writing.
- You are likely to have identified problem solving as a strength of reflection-in-action, whereas limited consciousness of the learning achieved might have been a limitation. Similarly, too much thought might be a barrier to developing reflection-on-action into action. You may have considered the potential depth for reflection as a strength of the reflection models, but the time needed for this as a limitation. You may also have viewed the acknowledgement of feelings in some of the models and reflective cycles as a strength that helps to take feelings forward in more positive ways, but the simplicity of the reflective cycles might also encourage superficial examination of issues. You may have noticed that the biographical approach helped you to integrate your reflective learning better, but that this might also have been challenging in what you found out about yourself. You might also have thought about the importance of credible evidence on which to base changing practice.

Further reading

Bulman, C and Schutz, S (eds) (2008) *Reflective Practice in Nursing*, 4th edn. Oxford: Blackwell Scientific Publications.

Gibbs, G (1988) *Learning by Doing: A guide to teaching and learning methods.* Oxford: Oxford Polytechnic, Further Education Unit.

Johns, C (2013) *Becoming a Reflective Practitioner*, 4th edn. Chichester: John Wiley & Sons, Inc.

Taylor, B (2010) *Reflective Practice for Healthcare Professionals*, 3rd edn. Maidenhead: Open University Press.

These books offer in-depth explanations of some of the models and frameworks discussed in this chapter.

Chapter 5 Creating space for reflection

NMC Standards of Proficiency for Registered Nurses

This chapter will address the following platforms and proficiencies:

Platform 5: Leading and managing nursing care and working in teams

5.9   Demonstrate the ability to challenge and provide constructive feedback about care delivered by others in the team and support them to identify and agree individual learning needs.

Platform 6: Improving safety and quality of care

6.9   Work with people, their families, carers and colleagues to develop effective improvement strategies for quality and safety, sharing feedback and learning from positive outcomes and experiences, mistakes and adverse outcomes and experiences.

6.11 Acknowledge the need to accept and manage uncertainty and demonstrate an understanding of strategies that develop resilience in self and others.

Chapter aims

After reading this chapter you will be able to:

- define the concept of transitional space;
- identify some barriers and limitations to reflection and strategies for overcoming these;
- examine the kinds of relationships that exist between people and how these might be more caring and compassionate;
- consider how you negotiate your position within healthcare;
- identify what makes spaces compelling for reflection and learning.

Introduction

Scenario 5.1: George

George had worked for some years as a registered nurse on a neurological ward where he had nursed Ms Gillespie. Ms Gillespie had, at that time, been newly diagnosed with a brain tumour and was admitted for investigations and to stabilise her on medication. At first Ms Gillespie was very emotional and confided in George that, as she, too, had been a nurse and knew what was in store for her, she didn't want to live with any handicap and be a burden to her long-time partner. Some time later, Ms Gillespie was admitted again with quite a severe hemiplegia, hemianopia and dysphagia. She recognised George and became quite emotional on seeing him. It surprised and relieved George somewhat to see that Ms Gillespie indicated that she was content and seemed to have found a level of acceptance of her condition and that George could still make Ms Gillespie laugh.

A few years later George was working night duty with the community's palliative care team and was allocated a client whose name rang a faint bell. When he arrived at the address, it turned out to be Ms Gillespie, who had been assigned care as she was nearing the end of her life. Ms Gillespie was sufficiently aware to recognise George and he could see that she was pleased to see him. Ms Gillespie's partner, Ms Tucker, seemed worn down and non-communicative, and George could only guess that the years and strain of Ms Gillespie's illness had left their mark on her and on their relationship. George was assigned a number of shifts and on the eighth morning at the end of his shift, Ms Gillespie took his hand and, with tears in her eyes, said that they would not see each other again because she felt sure that she would die before the day was out. On the way home, George felt uneasy and sad at leaving Ms Gillespie in this way because he felt that they had developed a bond over the years. That evening, George was called by the palliative care team's coordinator to say that Ms Gillespie had, indeed, died that afternoon.

Activity 5.1   Reflection

Take a moment to reflect on Scenario 5.1 about George and Ms Gillespie and you might find that a number of questions arise for you. For example, what do you think of the way in which the service user seemed to reset her boundaries as her illness progressed? What could the potential challenges be in supporting Ms Gillespie and her partner, Ms Tucker? Try to put yourself in George's position; how would you feel about this situation? Where do you think you could have the most beneficial reflection?

This is your own reflection, but an outline answer has been included at the end of the chapter.

The scenario above illustrates how nurses are sometimes confronted by situations where people's reactions can resonate with emotions and uncertainties they themselves are experiencing. Finding the time or a suitable place for reflection can be difficult. Often it is easy to find other things to put in its place, maybe because what reflection reveals makes you feel uncomfortable. Yet it is precisely continuing with familiar and comfortable ways of thinking and doing things that keeps you from exploring alternatives and considering change. Transition means moving from one position, or point of view, to another, and it is this shift between positions that can feel uncomfortable and uncertain. As you progress through your nursing programme, or even your career, more is expected from you in terms of knowledge, skills and decision-making.

This chapter introduces the concept of reflection as a *transitional space* in which you are encouraged to explore, develop and grow. The chapter considers some of the barriers and limitations to reflection and strategies you can use to overcome these. The chapter also asks you to examine the relationships that exist between individuals, and how you negotiate your place in diverse healthcare settings and situations. Finally, the chapter explores care and compassion for yourself and others, and what makes spaces compelling for reflection and learning.

Finding the time and space for reflection

Finding the time and space for reflection requires interest, motivation and commitment, as has been discussed in the previous chapters. Taylor (2010) suggests that reflection should be undertaken daily. Making reflection a part of your routine means that you are more likely to continue with it, and be able to see trends and changes taking place in both your practice and learning. This view suggests that, just as in Activity 5.1, space for reflection can be found at some point in the day. However, spaces for reflection in daily practice frequently appear at the margins of activity and are necessarily often brief and hurried in terms of the time used. Consider Scenario 5.2 to help you to identify where such spaces might appear in both personal and professional life.

Scenario 5.2: After hours with George

After leaving Ms Gillespie, George cycled home, showered, had some breakfast and went to bed to sleep for the day. Sleeping was fitful and so, when the phone rang at 18.30 and it was the palliative care team's coordinator to say that Ms Gillespie had died at 16.00, it somehow wasn't that much of a shock for George – somehow, he had been expecting it. George called friends to meet them in the pub later and went off for an hour's run along the beach. The pub with friends was great fun as it turned out to be a karaoke evening and everyone was keen to have a turn with the microphone. It was late to bed for George that night.

Activity 5.2   Reflection

Which activities could have offered George possibilities for reflection?

*   Try now to write down how you deal with situations that you find distressing. What strategies do you use to reach closure?

There is an outline answer to this question at the end of the chapter.

Through this scenario you may have identified that there is scope and space for reflection. It is, however, a person's focus, willingness and commitment to reflect that are necessary to maximise their learning. When time is limited, other priorities take over and it becomes difficult to maintain the discipline required for reflecting on your own learning in different situations both inside and outside the classroom and in practice.

One way to help maintain reflection is to use supporting elements, such as reflecting with others, either in groups or choosing a critical friend, who can help to invite commitment and provide additional support (Bulman and Schutz, 2008). Such support makes it easier to face and deal with the changes that reflection inevitably brings. Peer support is an important part of reflection in that it offers the opportunity for a two-way process of learning from the dialogue (Johns, 2007). Such dialogue involves reflective telling as well as reflective receiving. For example, when discussing how you feel with someone else they are likely to ask you what sparked that emotion, which will stimulate you to reflect on some of the surrounding reasons and issues. Equally, your listener may then think about your reasoning and offer some of their own after reflecting on what you have said. In this way, reflection is mutually beneficial. In Scenario 5.1 the transition being experienced by Ms Gillespie and her partner resonated with George's uncertainties of emotional boundaries as a nurse. The reflective questioning in George's example was primarily internal and it might have been helpful for George to share his thoughts with a colleague or, in the case of a student nurse, with their practice supervisor.

For any nurse, it is important to recognise that practice is complex, constantly evolving and full of surprises. This means that it is essential for self-reflection to be a part of everyday practice (Crabtree, 2003). Therefore, peer-reflective dialogue needs to be recognised as a normal part of professional practice. Although we might realise the importance of peer-reflective dialogue from a theoretical perspective, we often do not take the time to initiate or engage with colleagues to discuss our experiences. We might think that this moment of contemplation is necessary only for the inexperienced, but nothing could be further from the truth. We proceed now to consider the kind of space created by the act of reflection.

Transitional space

Transitional space is, as the name suggests, a place where a person is in the throes of change. Jarvis (2006) identifies that learning means people move from a position of being to one of becoming. This means that, in the process of such adjustment, a person enters into a transitional space where there are a number of possibilities for their development, which need to be negotiated, and where they may become changed as people. For example, you will have entered your nurse preparation programme with an idea of who you are, but during the course this may start to shift as you 'become' a nurse. Similarly, if you are an experienced practitioner you will have an idea of the kind of practitioner you are. Nevertheless, as you gather experience you will 'become' more expert, maybe a manager, a nurse specialist, an advanced practitioner or a nurse educator.

Transitional space, originally conceptualised by Winnicott (1965), is also defined as the point where subjective inner experience interacts with objective outer experience (Andrew et al., 2009; Hunt and West, 2007). For example, George was faced with an emotive situation in which Ms Gillespie shared awareness of her transition. For George, each contact with Ms Gillespie over the years, and in their final moment of farewell, meant that he was also experiencing transition (a) in his relationship with the service-user, (b) in needing to realign his emotionality with the external cues provided by Ms Gillespie and her partner, and (c) by learning to deal with his own emotions and 'reinterpret' them in terms of what he interpreted as 'professional behaviour'. The transitional space of learning is framed by how organisations and individuals, who help to create such a space, perceive themselves and interact. The following case study is provided as an example to help illustrate these processes.

Case study: Ellen's experience of failure

Ellen was at the end of the first year of her nursing programme and had recently received exam results that required her to retake the exam. The classes had been difficult to concentrate on, and Ellen acknowledged that she did not like the subject of clinical science. She had done well with her other subjects and was a good communicator.

Ellen was devastated because she felt she had worked really hard. There was very limited feedback to guide her about where she had gone wrong. Her first thought was that too much was expected of the student. She also felt angry towards the tutor, who she felt had not explained things well enough. Ellen was tempted to quit the programme because this felt so impossible. Gradually, as her anger and emotional response subsided, Ellen started thinking about what she could do. Her friend Mitch, who had passed the exam, told her she would be mad to quit now because she had almost passed the first year. He offered to help Ellen with her revising.

When Mitch and Ellen were revising it became obvious that Ellen had focused on a number of body systems in too much depth, and had not revised the learning outcomes for the module. Her knowledge of those particular systems was good and therefore she did have a reasonable knowledge that could be built on. Ellen started to feel less stupid and more in control of what she was doing. She could visualise herself as a nurse again and thoughts of quitting vanished. Ellen had also learned that her study technique needed adjusting. By focusing on the learning outcomes of the module, she could be more confident of achieving what was necessary to pass the exam. Ellen had learned a valuable lesson, namely how to deal with disappointment and still keep going. She became more resilient to adversity as a result.

This case study and scenarios demonstrate that transitional space is a place where we learn and develop, sometimes in painful ways, from how we deal with different situations and also that, as a result, we become changed as people. It is through constantly reviewing the interaction between our subjective experience and the feedback from the external world that we can develop. The external world relates to the people we interact with and the circumstances we have to deal with. By undertaking Activity 5.3 you will be able to identify where transitional space might be located within your own life and how you are learning and changing as a person.

Activity 5.3   Reflection

Try to remember a time of significant change or learning in your life and answer the following questions:

- What were the circumstances?
- How did you feel at the time?
- What did you learn?
- What change was brought about?
- Have you changed as a person as a result of the event?
- How did what you learned influence the change?
- Have you noticed any further changes, and when and where have these occurred?

There is an outline answer to this activity at the end of the chapter.

This activity is likely to have focused on personal circumstances, on how you have developed as a person before and during your nursing programme (and subsequent to it if you are an experienced practitioner), and on learning. Learning in different ways from those you are used to is, itself, a transitional space because you are challenged to adjust your subjective meaning of what is being asked. Having identified where transitional spaces have appeared in your own life, we now proceed to consider what might be some of the barriers and limitations to being able to reflect and learn in such spaces.

Barriers and limitations to reflection

Although reflection offers an opportunity for students and experienced practitioners to develop their own learning, it may become inhibited by certain challenges. Some of the difficulties that may create barriers to reflection include:

- not knowing how to reflect: you get stuck with how things feel and cannot make sense of things;
- tiredness: too much effort is required to maintain mental focus;
- lack of time: life gets in the way;
- not realising that reflection and learning can occur subconsciously and may result in the reinforcement of 'negative' ideas;
- lack of insight: it is difficult to recognise how personal actions might affect others;
- distractions: it is difficult to find a quiet space;
- lack of motivation: you cannot see the relevance of reflection;
- finding it difficult to deal with the consequences of reflection: reflection is too painful or revealing.

Even when you can engage in reflection, there may be factors that lead to limitations in the reflection achieved. According to Smith and Jack (2005), these constitute the following:

- Learning styles: some learning styles are likely to help you engage with reflection more readily and in more meaningful ways than others.
- It is not always easy for practitioners to articulate the knowledge they have; you may not be able to discern the decision-making thoughts of your supervisors.
- Not having evidence-based up-to-date knowledge.
- Reflection may be used for instrumental purposes and discontinued: reflection may remain focused on a course requirement, limiting you to a specific way of thinking.

Some of these aspects relate to personal knowledge of what reflection is about and what your role is within the process. Such barriers can be remedied by deepening your knowledge of reflection through reading. Other issues, such as having the time and space for reflection, can be overcome through organisation and negotiation which, in themselves, take effort and motivation. Ideally, taking the steps to overcome the barriers would come from realising that this is an opportunity to design your own learning. Limitations to reflection are likely to relate to the depth of reflection achieved. When reflection is a superficial or unconscious process, which may follow a reflection cycle without really ana-lysing what is happening and why, then it remains limited (Loughran, 2002).

Another way of overcoming some of the barriers and limitations to reflection is to ask a colleague or practice supervisor to help you with reflective processing. This means being able to share your thinking and meaning making with someone else in a way that debates and discusses your thinking as something that is developing, as illustrated in Scenario 5.1. This can be exposing in what it reveals of your 'becoming' to others, but is an important part of demonstrating progression and articulating how you are apply-ing your knowledge in different situations. Consideration of how you might do this in diverse healthcare settings now follows.

Negotiating your place in diverse healthcare settings

A key aspect of 'becoming' is through negotiating your position in diverse healthcare set-tings. This takes place through developing your role and idea of who you need to be in different arenas. For example, the role of the nurse in an accident and emergency (A&E) department will be very different from that of a nurse working in a mental health, pae-diatric, learning disability or community setting. In A&E, the nurse's role is focused on problem solving (usually as quickly as possible). In other settings the nurse will be working collaboratively with the patient and this may take longer. Although you are likely to be car-ing and empathetic in all situations, you may need to be more assertive in A&E, which will bring about a different development. Part of the process of negotiating your position is to understand your role relevant to your stage of preparation within the particular setting, and in relation to the nurse's role within the multiprofessional healthcare team. This involves:

- preparing for entering into the new setting: identifying key care priorities of the setting and getting to know the potential learning opportunities;
- being aware of ongoing changes and embracing these and the opportunities they offer;
- reflecting on your current knowledge: mapping your knowledge to that of the care priorities of the setting and planning to address any deficits, possibly through drafting a *learning contract* if you are a student;
- reflecting on what you are doing, the feedback you are getting and how you might see yourself developing, while you are in the care setting;
- summarising what you have learned about the care setting and yourself;
- reflecting on how any knowledge you have gained might be applicable in different settings.

Preparation, reflecting and summarising are important features in helping us to make sense of developing meaning from different settings. Undertaking Activity 5.4 will pro-vide you with the opportunity to apply and think about some of these issues in relation to your own experiences, in order to develop learning from those experiences.

Activity 5.4   Reflection

Consider the different placements you have had (or if you are an experienced practitioner the different positions you have held). How did you:

- prepare for the placement or role?
- experience change?
- identify others' expectations of you?
- understand your position in the setting?
- develop your learning in the setting?
- develop your identity?
- feel when you left the setting and why did you feel that way?
- plan what to do next?

As this activity is based on your own experiences, there is no outline answer at the end of the chapter.

You may have identified that you left some settings with a more positive feeling than others. By working through how you prepared to enter the setting, reflecting on what you learned and your developing identity while you were there, you can connect the past with the present and a potential future. This is an important part of negotiating your position in a transitional space.

The second aspect of negotiating your position relates to the levels of dependence, independence and interdependence that you may adopt, or be allowed to take on, in your working. When negotiating our position, previous experiences, as highlighted in Chapter 3, can influence our perceptions of others and ourselves (Andrew et al., 2009; Hunt and West, 2007). This may result in projecting the role of parent on to the supervisor, which can distort some of our responses. This process is illustrated within Scenario 5.3.

Scenario 5.3: Ravi's experience of two practice supervisors

Ravi was at the start of the third year of his nurse preparation programme and was working on a ward that specialised in diabetes. He had to return to this ward because he had to make up placement time he had lost due to sickness. While on this placement he was due to complete an assessment. His practice supervisor, Sylvia, had been quite critical about his performance during his previous placement. Sylvia was again his practice supervisor and Ravi felt very apprehensive because she had asked to have a formal meeting with him.

During their discussion, Sylvia commented that Ravi was still not meeting her expectations of his assessment objectives. She went through these in detail and identified that Ravi needed constant guidance. At this stage Sylvia was expecting that Ravi should be able to organise the care of a number of patients and hand over to others independently. She was concerned about whether Ravi was going to be able to pass the assessment and told him he needed to become more proactive in his dealings with patients and staff.

Ravi tried to explain that he knew what to do but wanted to confirm that this was correct. On leaving the meeting with Sylvia, Ravi felt demoralised and not sure what he could do to improve. He felt that everything he did was wrong. Ravi was due to work with another supervisor for the next two weeks as Sylvia was on leave.

Ravi met with his new practice supervisor, Wendy, on the Monday of the following week. Wendy explained which patients she wanted Ravi to look after and organise the care for, and asked Ravi to tell her what he saw as the main priorities. Intermittently Wendy would join Ravi for aspects of care such as the drug round, or when the consultant needed to see a patient, or during handover. She allowed Ravi to give the main information and would add points as necessary. By the end of the first week Ravi's confidence had grown. He began to think that he could pass this assessment because Wendy told him he was working more independently. On the last week of his placement Sylvia was not available, so Wendy undertook Ravi's assessment. Although there were a few areas in which she suggested he could develop further, Wendy was satisfied that Ravi had passed his assessment.

Activity 5.5   Reflection

* In what ways were Ravi's responses distorted? What else could he have done to help in negotiating his position?

There are outline answers to these questions at the end of the chapter.

As is noted in this scenario, the quality of interactions can have a profound effect on our responses and ability to learn. When we are treated in what we perceive to be negative ways, we may also respond less confidently. Part of creating spaces for reflection includes using care and compassion when doing so in order to create a meaningful space for learning. We proceed now to consider issues relating to care and compassion within spaces of reflection.

Care and compassion

Care and compassion in terms of learning relate to how cared for you feel yourself to be. Although the 6 Cs were developed for nurses caring for patients, we should also be extending these to how we interact with each other. Nursing practice can sometimes be so hectic that you barely have time to think, so you feel under constant pressure. Creating space for reflection is a form of care that allows you to take stock of what is happening and grasp the opportunity to learn. Creating space for yourself to reflect is a form of self-caring that enables you to come to a different view of yourself (Schmidt, 2008). Equally, biographical construction and reflection, as discussed in Chapter 3, have the potential to change impressions and develop your learning in more affirming ways that are compassionate. The ability to explore the self is an important element of self-caring (Chan and Schwind, 2006). Undertaking Activity 5.6 might help you to read situations differently and see the opportunities for becoming self-caring.

Activity 5.6   Critical thinking

Look again at the case study of Ellen's failure (pages 92–3) and Scenario 5.3, Ravi's experience of two practice supervisors, and consider the following:

- Who showed care and compassion?
- How were care and compassion demonstrated, if at all?
- What were the results for Ellen and Ravi?
- What did they take forward from their situations?
- If care and compassion are absent, what is, or is likely to be, the outcome?
- How can we show care and compassion for ourselves and others as part of reflection?

There are outline answers to this activity at the end of the chapter.

Activity 5.7   Reflection

When you have completed answering the above points, write a reflective summary of what you have learned using the pro forma from Chapter 1 (page 27), and include an action plan for how you can show care and compassion. Please use this action plan to work towards the goals you have set yourself and reflect on your learning as you progress.

As this activity is based on your learning experience, there is no outline answer at the end of the chapter.

Through undertaking Activity 5.7, you are likely to have viewed the situations in more positive and affirmative ways. Reading situations from such a perspective can help to open a space that is more compelling for learning, not in a coercive sense, but by being open-minded and engaged. We proceed now to consider such a space for reflection and learning, which draws all the parts already discussed into a whole.

Space that is compelling for reflection and learning

Space might be described as a *compelling space* (Horowitz, 2004, p155), where people initiate opportunities by engaging with each other to learn something new. Such acts of initiation might relate to either you choosing whether or not to reflect, and so learn, or to the design that you give to your reflection. In other words, do you choose to reflect with others, in written form or by thinking things through on your own? A compelling space is one that invites meaningful learning and is where people feel able to acknowledge that they do not know (Howatson-Jones, 2010). In such a space you are empowered to become proactive in developing curiosity, enquiry and meaning. It is here that real autonomy may be found in how you develop your own knowledge and take control of your learning. To do this you need to integrate the personal with the professional, as outlined in Chapter 3, and so create a compelling space. In Scenario 5.1 George recognises such autonomy by allowing himself to reflect on his relationship with Ms Gillespie and how the situation impacts on his way of being. This illustrates how we can take more control of our own transitions to become a qualified nurse or within the context of life-long learning. The following case study offers an example of how a compelling space is created.

Case study: Jared's experience of a compelling space

Jared was at the end of his nursing programme and was working in an ambulatory cancer care centre. He really enjoyed this placement because there did not seem to be any hierarchical distinctions between the medical and the nursing staff. They all worked as a team in a person-centred way. A poem written by one of the patients was displayed in the colourful waiting area and seemed to sum up these impressions in the words used. Jared looked at this poem every day when he came on duty and it inspired him. Before finishing the placement his practice supervisor, Abby, asked Jared to share his reflections and learning with the team. Inspired by the poem and the person-centred attitude of the team, Jared began with the poem that had so inspired him and his reflections emanating from this and his observations of the team

(Continued)

(Continued)

and his learning about person-centredness. The team gave Jared positive feedback. He left the placement feeling affirmed and valued. When writing his reflective diary at home that night he considered what had helped his learning. It was a mix of the positive atmosphere, the team working together, the inspiration of the poem that had motivated him and the team's feedback on his practice. All these combined to make the space compelling for his learning.

Chapter summary

This chapter has introduced the concept of transitional space and offered you the opportunity to examine some transitional spaces in your own life through the activities provided. By exploring some of the barriers and limitations to reflection, suggestions for how to overcome these have also been illuminated and can be employed to help you increase your reflective opportunities. By examining how you negotiate your place within diverse healthcare settings, issues of care and compassion have been raised in how these influence the quality of the learning experience. By empowering individuals, compelling spaces for learning and reflection are created. Chapter 6 continues this theme by looking at reflection and reflexivity.

Activities and scenarios: Brief outline answers

Activity 5.1 Reflection (page 89)

Places that you might have identified as being potentially available for reflection could have been:

- while eating breakfast – contemplating your current knowledge base in a new setting;
- while cycling – consider what information you want/need to find out;
- while exercising – combining physical and mental activity by revisiting new knowledge while doing repetitive exercises;
- while out with friends – through being in the midst of life and fun you would be placing life and death in perspective and realising that, as a nurse and even though you have an affection for a service user or their carer, you cannot carry the/their whole world on your shoulders.

You might not have taken up these particular opportunities for reflection because of a lack of time, or because you wanted to do something else, or because you were tired;

however, these suggestions could help you to combine everyday activities with reflective moments.

Activity 5.2 Scenario 5.1 After hours with George (page 91)

You might have considered the following activities as offering scope for reflection:

- undertaking systematic reflection using a recognised model as discussed in Chapter 4;
- talking about practice with others: reflecting on observed practice and how this compared with knowledge;
- talking about the day with others: identifying emotions and highlighting positives and areas for further reflection;
- working with an expert/specialist: reflecting on differences between settings.

Activity 5.3 Reflection (page 93)

In considering the question about significant change in your life, you might have thought about when you were an adolescent, or maybe when you became a parent for the first time. Some of the feelings evoked are likely to have been anxiety and uncertainty. You might have learned new skills and this in turn may have helped you to grow in confidence. You are likely to have become increasingly independent and able to make decisions for yourself. Modifications to this change are likely to have ensued from problems you encountered and successes you experienced, so that there will have been further uncertain times, but also greater ability to direct your progression.

Activity 5.5 Scenario 5.3: Ravi's experience of two practice supervisors (page 97)

Ravi's previous experience on the ward, working with Sylvia, had been anxiety provoking because of the way that he perceived her constant criticism of him. Therefore, he was adopting a child's role of waiting to be told what to do in order to get things right. He perceived Sylvia in a parent's role of knowing best. With Wendy, Ravi was able to gradually move to a more grown-up role and perceived that he had the space to make decisions, but that Wendy was still available should he come across anything he did not understand or of which was not sure. This situation will be recognisable as a student or as a qualified healthcare professional – you will always encounter people who trigger this kind of response. Ideally, Ravi should have spoken to Sylvia about their working relationship and negotiated how they could move forward. This might be difficult to do but it does show the characteristics of a professional; it takes courage and commitment (two of the 6 Cs) to address a situation where you feel vulnerable. If he felt unsure, Ravi could have spoken to the university tutor about his experience as a way of helping him to negotiate his position and prepare for the meeting. He could also have asked the university tutor to chair the meeting with Sylvia and, in so doing, would create a learning situation for himself and Sylvia – a situation in which he would be able to ask the tutor for feedback on his communication and interaction strategies and, consequently, be appropriate for Ravi, a final-year student nurse. We should remain mindful that dealing with difficult or sensitive issues, as this example shows, takes practice and confidence. It is, therefore, wise to start practising from the beginning of your programme so that, by the time you get to Year 3, you have built the necessary confidence and techniques. At this point, you are advised to read the Section *Practise efficiently: Work cooperatively* of the NMC's Code (NMC, 2018b) which deals with appropriate referral of care to colleagues, and inter- and intraprofessional communication to ensure safety and quality of care (items 8.1–8.6).

Activity 5.6 Critical thinking (page 98)

Your answers might have included the following.

- You might have identified that Mitch showed care and compassion towards Ellen in the case study, and Wendy showed care and compassion in her working with Ravi in the scenario.
- Care and compassion were demonstrated by Mitch in helping Ellen to revise, and by Wendy in supervising Ravi at key points in his work to ensure that he was not undermined but supported.
- Ellen was able to adjust her study and revision techniques, and Ravi was able to function in a more independent way.
- Ellen had become more resilient to adversity and Ravi could see himself as a capable practitioner.
- In the absence of care and compassion, people feel diminished and less capable, and are more liable to make mistakes.
- Showing care and compassion for ourselves involves getting to know ourselves better through some of the techniques suggested in this book. Showing care and compassion for others involves looking for positives rather than being critical in negative ways.

Further reading

Honey, P and Mumford, A (2006) *The Learning Styles Questionnaire: 80 item version.* Maidenhead: Peter Honey.

This book explains different learning styles and offers the opportunity for identifying your own learning style.

Jarvis, P (2006) *Towards a Comprehensive Theory of Human Learning: Lifelong learning and the learning society,* Vol 1. London: Routledge.

This book offers a broad examination of different types of learning and is helpful for understanding how and why we learn.

Johns, C (2007) Deep in reflection. *Nursing Standard*, 21(38): 24–5.

This article explores the mutual benefits of reflecting with others.

Useful websites

BBC Key Skills: **www.bbc.co.uk/keyskills/extra/module1/1.shtml**

This website identifies different ways of learning relating to key skills.

BBC Learning Styles: **www.open2.net/survey/learningstyles**

This website offers another view of learning styles and includes an online survey to help you determine your style.

Chapter 6 Reflection and reflexivity

NMC Standards of Proficiency for Registered Nurses

This chapter will address the following platforms and proficiencies:

Platform 1: Being an accountable professional

1.17 Take responsibility for continuous self-reflection, seeking and responding to support and feedback to develop their professional knowledge and skills.

Platform 5: Leading and managing nursing care and working in teams

5.6 Exhibit leadership potential by demonstrating an ability to guide, support and motivate individuals and interact confidently with other members of the care team.

5.10 Contribute to supervision and team reflection activities to promote improvements in practice and services.

Chapter aims

After reading this chapter you will be able to:

- describe reflective conceptualisation at different stages of professional preparation;
- demonstrate how reflexivity may change your awareness in new ways;
- identify developing insight;
- relate to the experiences of others.

Introduction

Scenario 6.1: Boris's experience of sharing work

Boris was in the final year of his nursing programme. He was completing his dissertation and this week the tutor had asked the class to share their work at the last session so that all could benefit from this learning. Boris was worried about doing this because he normally kept all his work private to avoid accidental or intentional plagiarism or collusion. During the mid-morning break Boris voiced his concerns to some of his peers. Some were sympathetic to his views whereas others reacted in a more hostile way, saying Boris was assuming that some of the class were dishonest. This led to an argument and Boris went home after class in a bad mood.

That evening, after he had calmed down, Boris decided to reflect on the morning session and the argument that ensued. Boris felt protective of his work because his final degree classification was important to him and he did not want it jeopardised through academic mistakes at this late stage. Analysing this Boris became aware that his family had always had a strong work ethic in all they did; his siblings had taken on after-school jobs as well as gaining excellent exam results leading to good careers; this had clearly influenced him. He wanted his mother, in particular, to be proud of his final degree result because she had worked so hard after his father died when he was 2 years old. Boris then considered how the reasons for his reluctance to share his work might have appeared to others. He realised that he had assumed that some of his peers might use the work for their own gain without any evidence. For a previous assignment, Boris had been tempted to cut and paste some useful information from the internet, but had heeded his lecturer's constant warnings about academic theft and completed his own search and referenced correctly. Boris realised that it was this ethical wavering that was the basis for his views.

Boris prepared for the last session by identifying the reasons for his choice of topic, how he went about finding the information and what implications for practice had emerged. He shared the overview and summary with the class and found their questions helpful. Some of his peers in turn identified how useful they found Boris's method for searching for information. By doing this last session Boris had a much better grasp of his dissertation subject and was able to complete writing it. Boris changed his view about the usefulness of sharing information and work.

The example offered in Scenario 6.1 illustrates how our upbringing and personal responses can influence our thinking about situations and the people involved in them. By reflecting on this we can modify our behaviour, enabling deeper learning, as well as having the potential to influence others. As you progress through your programme, you will also develop resources and skills that enable you to direct and modify some of your experiences. Taking ownership of situations and what is being learned empowers you to consider alternatives and to make changes.

This chapter begins by defining what reflexivity is, and then proceeds to offer opportunities for you to examine how you can influence your experiences and how those experiences might influence you. The focus is on the role of reflexivity in developing opportunities for learning.

What is reflexivity?

In the previous chapters we have discussed reflection and reflective practice and, although reflection can be seen as a way of being – a way to learn from experience through asking questions – reflexivity is to turn back on yourself. Hertz (1997, p viii) suggests that it is like having *an ongoing conversation about experience while simultaneously living in the moment.* This is clearly illustrated in the story in Scenario 6.1, in which where Boris felt restricted in fully participating in the group process. This was not a conscious distrust of his peers or unwillingness to share his ideas or contribute to the group process. Rather, his behaviour was influenced by his personal autobiography (as we discussed in Chapter 3). This required Boris to examine the surrounding factors of how situations arise and in what ways his reflections might help him to influence his experiences, as well as how those experiences might shape him as a person and a practitioner.

Reflexivity, therefore, involves a continuous review of personal action to enact change (Alheit and Dausien, 2007). To do this requires you to examine your personal actions and assumptions within the context of wider social interactions. For example, you are a developing practitioner within a wider profession, which has rules and regulations and expectations of its practitioners, but is also represented by those practitioners. In this way it becomes possible for you to open up opportunities to consider how you are influencing your learning, how you are influencing professional understanding, and how this is also influenced by life and social patterns. For example, how you study for exams will in part be influenced by the ways you have found successful in the past, but also by how your peer group perceives the concept of studying. In Boris's example in Scenario 6.1, his background had influenced him to be self-reliant in his studying. He experienced an ethical dilemma but came back on track because of fear of the penalties, but this experience has created assumptions about others. It is only through reflecting reflexively that Boris comes to a different conclusion that benefits his learning positively.

Equally, part of reflexivity is recognising that knowledge and knowing are integrated with the self. In other words, knowing is not separate from you as a person and what you bring to your understanding at a given time. For example, the culture you grew up in will have been influential in shaping who you are and how you perceive things, as discussed in Chapter 3 and Scenario 6.1. This is part of a *socialisation* process that continues throughout life (Jarvis, 2007). Culture and socialisation may influence your perceptions of what is similar to your view, what is different and what is classified as important. This will have been modified by other cultures such as school and working life. The professional culture and contexts of nursing will continue to alter your sense of self and how you integrate knowledge and knowing. Socialisation into the profession and its body of knowledge sets boundaries that start to become defended when working with others (Ousey and Johnson, 2007). Anxiety, fear and overemphasis on results can lead to focusing on a tick-box approach to the completion of learning tasks, but not on actually accomplishing learning. Reflexivity, as a consequence, can therefore become limited and superficial when other priorities take over. In Scenario 6.1, Boris is initially held back by such an attitude. Reflexivity involves 'mindfulness', which means paying attention to situations, staff conduct and practice contexts to monitor for potential problems and solutions (Iedema, 2011).

Consider Scenario 6.2 to identify how reflexivity may become limited between teams.

Scenario 6.2: Sue's experience of fragmenting teams

Sue was in the second year of her nursing programme and working on an orthopaedic ward. The ward next door was often short-staffed, and the qualified nurses from Sue's ward were frequently asked to cover. Staff on Sue's ward helped each other out by coming in earlier or going home later. They were resentful that the ward next door did not seem to do the same and that they often had to help them. Sue observed that this started to affect relationships and cause tensions. The hostile atmosphere also affected opportunities to learn.

Sue observed that, on her ward, there were numerous opportunities for learning because the staff constantly shared practice and reflected on what they were doing. The ward manager had set up a programme of lunchtime sessions where they could do this, and this included other professionals who came in to talk about their perspectives as well. However, it was interesting that the staff did not appear to be reflecting on the relationship with the other ward and Sue started to think about why this might be.

It seemed that there were different cultures on the two different wards. On Sue's ward, the manager was very proactive in trying to support learning and her staff. On the other ward, staff felt that they had little say in their working life and seemed to experience less support. Sue came to this conclusion because one of her friends was working on the other ward. Sue wondered whether the perceived lack of support was why staff were reluctant to give up any more of their own time and whether this was contributing to the atmosphere between the wards.

(Continued)

(Continued)

Sue considered the difference in attitude between the wards in terms of being a nurse and what this meant to her. She had come into nursing because she saw helping people as a vocation rather than a job. To Sue, this meant that, if patients needed some extra time, it might require her staying behind beyond the end of a shift. Having been brought up to help people, Sue saw this as a normal part of her role. She felt she could understand the resentment of the staff on her ward, because she perceived the other ward's staff not contributing as much and sometimes taking advantage as they knew they would get help.

Activity 6.1   Reflection

- Looking at this scenario reflexively, what other interpretations might you have? What area of commonality might offer the potential for the staff to forge a different relationship?

There are outline answers to these questions at the end of the chapter.

Scenario 6.2 might have helped you to identify that, even when we are reflecting, we often do not think reflexively about situations, how culture influences us and what this contributes to the circumstances we encounter.

By undertaking Activity 6.2 you will be able to develop some insight into how culture influences your reflexive thinking.

Activity 6.2   Critical thinking

When thinking about the different cultures you have experienced at home, at school, through your friends and professionally, consider the following questions.

- How have the various cultures influenced you?
- What is important to you in learning to be a nurse?
- How does your background influence your views of learning as a nurse?

- What kind of knowledge is important to you and why do you think it is important?
- How do you develop knowing?
- How has developing as a nurse professional affected the kind of knowledge you see as important?

There is an outline answer to this activity at the end of the chapter.

Through completing the activity, you may have identified some influences on the way in which you perceive things and what is important. In this way you can develop awareness of how your thinking is shaped and how you can start to exert some influence on modifying your thinking and circumstances. We proceed now to consider the process of taking ownership.

Taking ownership

Taking ownership means taking responsibility for your own action or inaction. In other words, in terms of reflection and reflexivity, this means being responsible for examining issues and being honest with yourself in what you contribute to the situation, and what the outcomes say about your approach. By recognising your own participation it will become clearer where adjustments might be needed, or might make the most contribution. The process of taking ownership involves:

- developing self-awareness;
- communicating developmental needs;
- using emotional intelligence;
- becoming historically and politically aware;
- informing yourself.

Personal insight and self-awareness are the cornerstones of reflexivity (Lee, 2009). Self-awareness relates to being attuned to what makes up the inner world (van Ooijen, 2013) – in other words, how you really think and feel about things, what values you might have, and any potential contradictions between what you say and what you do (Manley et al., 2011). Superficial approaches to reflection and reflexivity are sometimes used as ways of avoiding ownership, because their instrumental purpose and limited analysis circumvent challenging the *self-concept*, and also, therefore, do not result in any lasting change. The practitioner who has developed personal insight and self-awareness will internalise these characteristics to become their way of being. Consequently, in order to continue their learning, they will remain alert as to how others react to their interventions. Communication is, therefore, the key; it is vitally important to check whether your perceptions are accurate, and to explore the best way to move forward.

Although communicating your developmental needs to others is part of the skills set you need to build up during your nursing programme, this remains a life-long learning process. As nurses, we are expected to be self-aware about our knowledge and competence, and to address any deficits (NMC, 2018a). It is through reflection that such deficits will come to light in meaningful ways for you, even if they were highlighted by others, such as your practice supervisor or a colleague. You learn communication skills as part of your nurse preparation programme, first by looking at basic theories in the first year and then by learning how to apply these in different settings throughout the rest of the programme. Nursing communication needs to be both therapeutic and professional in relation to how you communicate with patients, families and carers, but also with other professionals when organising care (Sully and Dallas, 2010). However, communicating your (learning) needs is a part that might feel challenging when you lack confidence, or have concerns about how you are perceived by others. Even experienced practitioners might fear acknowledging developmental needs and this can leave you feeling very vulnerable. Taking ownership of your needs is an important aspect of being a nursing practitioner and requires:

- seeking appropriate support and guidance;
- dealing with your emotions constructively;
- acknowledging and embracing feelings of vulnerability and discussing these with a practice supervisor or colleague;
- addressing knowledge gaps;
- undertaking independent study.

Nursing involves dealing with service users and carers or family members who are often distressed or traumatised by their situation. Constant exposure to distressing situations can feel quite burdensome for the nurse or student nurse, and this is known as emotional labour. Emotional intelligence, on the other hand, is having awareness of one's own emotions and being able to read the emotional cues of others (Hurley and Linsley, 2012). When first starting your nursing preparation programme you may have been somewhat aware of your own emotional reactions but were possibly less proficient in reading those of others. As you develop through the programme you will find yourself understanding your own emotions better as you reflect on your reactions and behaviour in relation to your autobiography (as discussed in Chapter 3). Similarly, you will find that you are 'tuning in' to the emotional states of your clients and patients – in a way 'reading' people by recognising cues in their behaviour. In other words, these skills can be brought to reading situations reflectively by 'tuning in' to the emotional vibrations that resonate through the situation, and the language that you and others use to describe it. Using emotional intelligence means being able to distinguish stressors and work that is emotionally meaningful and how internal values are aligned with these (Price, 2008). At first, your reflection will almost certainly be triggered by emotion, but, unless emotional intelligence is activated to read the situation and people's reactions, reflection will remain bound to feelings and not move forward to actual learning. Part of such adjustment requires being aware of what has gone before in order to be alert to cues in the present – as previously mentioned this is a life-long learning activity that you will continue to hone and perfect. There will, however, be times that your 'reading' of the situation is inaccurate – remain mindful that this is not 'failure', but yet another opportunity to reflect and learn reflexively from the situation.

Historical insight is an important part of this process. For example, if you are aware that a particular unit has undergone considerable change in previous years, it will not surprise you to find that some staff may be resistant to further adaptations. Political changes have a profound effect on healthcare priorities and resources, and these are equally influential in how supported, or not, practitioners feel themselves to be. It is sometimes easy within reflection to make assumptions about situations and their solutions without a historical and political perspective, and where reflective solutions in reality are unworkable and therefore lead to further frustration. Part of guarding against this circumstance is to inform yourself of the background and context of the situation and some of the surrounding issues, and to ensure that your knowledge pertaining to these is up to date. Informing yourself may require some independent study and, consequently, time which will need to be factored into your learning plan. Consider the following scenario to identify processes of taking ownership of reflection and reflexivity.

Scenario 6.3: Geeta's experience of developing ownership in reflection

Geeta was in the final year of her nursing programme and working in an operating theatre environment. She was on her last extended placement and was hoping to secure a permanent post as a theatre nurse practitioner after qualifying. Geeta had been in this placement for five weeks when a second-year student, Joe, was also placed there for a shorter time, as part of his acute care experience. Geeta did not really get on with Joe because she found him rather patronising, and it appeared that some of the other staff also did not like him very much. Geeta's practice supervisor asked her to help orient Joe to the theatre suite and the ways of working, because she felt that Joe might respond more positively to another student.

Geeta found that Joe acted as if he was in charge because he tried to take over things that Geeta normally did. The patients seemed to like Joe, however, because he had a good patient manner that put them at ease when they arrived looking nervous. Joe tended to want to be in the thick of the most complicated cases and this sometimes limited Geeta's opportunities.

On this particular day Geeta and Joe were working in the same theatre. Geeta had helped set up the instrument trolley with her practice supervisor, and both she and Joe were now helping to set up the staff with their final requirements. The operation commenced and Geeta and Joe were invited to view the surgeon's actions more closely.

(Continued)

(Continued)

On turning round, Geeta noticed that Joe had accidentally touched part of the instrument trolley and potentially desterilised it. Geeta had no option but to tell the scrub nurse, which she attempted to do as discreetly as possible. However, the trolley needed to be changed and this caused a short delay that was noticeable to everyone.

After the operation was completed, Geeta was helping to clean up in the dirty area. When Geeta was alone, Joe came in and angrily told Geeta she had made him look really stupid and how dare she show him up. Geeta explained why it had been necessary to change the trolley. Joe replied that it was not up to her and she was getting above her place. At this point, feeling under attack, Geeta told Joe that she found his attitude difficult at times, a view shared by some of the staff. Joe grabbed a passing qualified nurse and asked her if this was true. The nurse replied that there were times when he appeared not to listen to people. Joe stormed out of the room.

Geeta had to take a short break because she felt very upset by this incident. On her way home that evening she started to reflect on the experience. Geeta was confident that she had taken the right action but was less sure about telling Joe that other staff found him difficult. She also wondered whether part of her reaction was due to her own difficulties with him.

Activity 6.3 Reflection

Please write down your answers to the following questions:

- If you were Geeta, how and where would you start to take ownership of this reflection?
- Which particular elements of the scenario would you draw on as being particularly important?
- Try to reflect on this scenario as broadly as possible. You might want to consider issues related to interpersonal communication, organisational structure, responsibility, status, autobiographies of those involved, etc.

There are outline answers to these questions at the end of the chapter.

This scenario might have helped you to think about your reflections using emotional intelligence to better discern the perspectives of others. Reflexivity means that we are able to judge the effects of our actions on others as much as the effects they may have on us. We proceed now to consider the role of reflexivity in developing learning.

Role of reflexivity in developing learning

The role of reflexivity in learning has been defined as how students or registered nurses orient themselves to learning opportunities (Cassidy, 2009). Such orientation involves bringing personal knowledge to the caring situation, at the same time as recognising what meaning is made from the situation and related knowledge. To do this requires:

- being aware of internal dialogue;
- embedding learning through integration;
- recognising the relatedness of knowledge;
- having awareness of nursing as a community of practice.

To be aware of an internal dialogue means listening to internal reasoning processes, meaning and decision-making. For example, you might be involved in an assessment discussion with your practice supervisor in which you are talking about how you communicate with patients. Your practice supervisor may highlight particular techniques that need to be used, but that you know how to use. You might identify that your meaning and your practice supervisor's interpretation of these techniques are at variance and that you need to decide how to proceed. Throughout the conversation you will be aware of a running internal commentary. Some call this commentary an internal practice supervisor (Percival, 2001) and this internal dialogue may either help or hinder the outcome of your deliberations, depending on how in harmony it is with, or how divergent it is from, your thinking and acting. This process is a part of integrating learning.

In Chapter 1 we briefly mentioned Carper's (1978) patterns of knowing and that integrating learning means drawing together these different strands of knowing and knowledge gained through the complex business of nursing and life in general (Zander, 2007). The integration process involves reflection, including listening for the internal commentary as explained above, in order to embed new information and connect it to the knowledge already in place. The connections are made through reflecting on what is brought to situations, what is taken away from them and how well things went. This is part of the process of integrating learning previously explained in Chapter 3. Imagining connects here to the internal dialogue that assesses possible consequences of actions. In this way knowledge starts to be related rather than simply accumulated.

Relating knowledge also makes it easier to apply it to different situations. For example, relating knowledge of different communication techniques makes it possible to understand how some might, for instance, be more applicable to a short-term setting than others. Equally, relating knowledge of physiological effects of virus invasion on the body to knowledge of economic and social pressures makes it easier to understand contrary behaviours and the prolongation of infection. Understanding the evolution of theories and concepts helps to develop a reflexive frame by which these may also be questioned. Theories are suppositions that develop learning when questioned through reflexive thinking. Without such questioning, theories remain dormant in terms of learning and, consequently, are not easily recalled or applied. Part of being a reflexive practitioner is to help develop theories through different applications within the community of nursing.

Nursing is part of a community of practice through sharing a common purpose of caring for people. People exist within a *community of practice* (Andrew et al., 2008) in the way they organise themselves and their lives. Nursing, as a community, offers the possibility for integrating practice with academic knowledge through providing engagement that questions both theory and practice (Andrew et al., 2008). As a developing nurse you embed learning in that community of practice through the ideas you reciprocally work through in your university programme, self-directed study and practice. The capacity to be reflexive within your community determines how successful this process is. Collaborating reflexively within a community of practice helps the student, and the practice supervisor, to learn both personally and as professionals. Sharing ideas in a community of practice helps all parties to develop and ensures that practice is dynamic rather than stagnating.

Consider Scenario 6.4 to identify processes of reflexive development of learning.

Scenario 6.4: Charmaine's reflexive learning experience

Charmaine was in the first placement of her second year of the nursing degree programme and was working in a supported housing complex with adults with moderate learning disabilities. Although Charmaine felt that she had developed good communication skills from her placement experience in the first year and the voluntary work she had done in the local care home before starting the programme, she was somewhat uncertain how these could be applied in a learning disability setting. This was discussed on the first day when Charmaine and her practice supervisor, Jerry, had their initial meeting. Jerry reassured Charmaine that for the first week he would be expecting her to observe and support the service users with activities of daily living while settling in to the new environment. Charmaine was not too concerned about the practical skills but was still apprehensive about communication with the service users because she wanted to ensure that she provided the people with choices and was able to communicate in an appropriate way. Charmaine observed how Jerry always had a laugh with the patients and the easy therapeutic relationship he established with them. She also observed how clear his explanations were for the patients and also for her when she asked about the use of different tools.

At the end of the first week Charmaine and Jerry reflected on the week's learning for both of them. Charmaine told Jerry what she had observed about his communication style. Jerry in turn highlighted how valuable he found Charmaine's presence for making him think about the explanation for what he was doing, and helping him to develop his teaching practice through sharing learning and knowledge. Charmaine was surprised by this because Jerry seemed so knowledgeable. His last statement that there was always something to learn made Charmaine think.

Activity 6.4   Reflection

- What reflexive learning is taking place here for Charmaine and Jerry?

There is an outline answer to this question at the end of the chapter.

Chapter summary

This chapter has begun to define reflexivity. By offering activities that ask the novice and developing nurse to consider how they employ reflexivity, the chapter has offered opportunities to make sense of internal dialogue and cultural considerations within the wider community of nursing. Through inclusion of examples of how to take ownership of reflective and reflexive processes and what they may reveal, the chapter has made it possible to develop real insight and increase self-awareness, and consequently the effectiveness of the practitioner. By underpinning this with developing emotional intelligence you have the possibility for reading situations more reflexively and integrating this knowledge differently to develop caring. The importance of this as a part of reflective practice will be continued in Chapter 7.

Activities and scenarios: Brief outline answers

Activity 6.1 Reflection (page 108)

Although Sue's background had laid the foundation for helping her to view nursing as a vocation, life circumstances for some people might also get in the way. Equally, nursing is a highly skilled profession that deserves to be remunerated. Both sets of staff appeared to feel coerced into working in a different way, provoking anxiety and making it more difficult for them to think reflexively. When thinking reflexively, Sue might see that, if the situation of helping out the ward next door continued indefinitely, they might never get the resources they needed in terms of extra staff because the staff shortages remain 'invisible' to middle and higher management. Perhaps this could offer a starting point for dialogue between the two wards, in how they might address this in the longer term together, and so develop a more positive relationship. Talking in this way might also help them to share practice and, through this, develop learning opportunities. You might also want to reflect on whose responsibility it should be to initiate this discussion between the wards: should it be the ward managers, or should this come from the staff nurses and other staff working on the ward? Try to question your answers as to why you think one thing or another. You might want to explore how the NMC's Code (NMC, 2018b) relates to this situation, for example, the section *Practise efficiently* (items 8.2, 8.4, 8.5, 8.7, 9.1, 9.2, 9.3 and 9.4) and the section *Promote professionalism and trust* (items 20.2, 20.3 and 20.8). It would be good to pause briefly here to image the potential consequences the fallout from this situation could have in terms of bullying and harassment.

Activity 6.2 Critical thinking (pages 108–9)

When completing the activity you might have highlighted some of the following points:

- Home and school are likely to have influenced your approach to studying and learning in more or less positive ways.
- Learning the skills of being a nurse is likely to be a priority for you.
- Your background may have given you a view of learning as a nurse that differs concerning practical and academic contributions.
- Practical knowledge may be of greater importance than academic knowledge, or scientific knowledge may be a greater priority than softer skills such as communication, because this is the evidence base for your actions.
- Your knowing is likely to develop by doing, as well as through sharing your practice and reflecting.
- Developing as a nurse professional is likely to have identified the importance of a variety of knowledge, spanning the psychological, sociological, biological, ethical, spiritual, personal and professional.

Activity 6.3 Reflection (page 112)

In Scenario 6.3, we should be mindful of the roles and responsibilities of Geeta, her practice supervisor, Joe and Joe's practice supervisor. Before addressing the actual situation that caused the escalation, Geeta could have been proactive in clarifying with her practice supervisor what her status and responsibility were with regard to Joe. This should have been discussed in a three-way meeting of Geeta, Joe and the practice supervisor. This could have provided Geeta with the authority to correct Joe and discuss his behaviour. Certainly, early in Joe's placement he might not have clearly understood the principles that need to be adhered to in an operating theatre. Part of Geeta's reflexive learning would be on how she had prepared Joe for his being in an operating theatre and what she would need to do in order to prevent this from happening again. In terms of the NMC's Code (NMC, 2018b) you might want to read the section *Practise effectively* (items 8.1–8.6 and 9.1–9.4).

First, Geeta should reflect on the relationship between her and Joe, and between Joe and the other staff.

Geeta also needs to consider their differing developmental needs and whether these have been adequately discussed with their practice supervisors, because it appears that their needs are being amalgamated and this is limiting Geeta's learning. This could have been clarified in the initial meeting if, for example, Geeta was Joe's practice supervisor as part of her own learning objectives.

Another area that Geeta might want to reflect on is her autobiography. Was she feeling jealous of Joe because, with his arrival, she was not getting all the attention from the staff? Was she envious that he was able to communicate so well with the patients and able to calm them? Is her response to Joe driven by feelings of power and was her response to Joe's mistake an opportunity to 'take him down a peg or two'?

Certainly, a substantial part of Geeta's reflection needs to consider her use of emotional intelligence. Is she aware of her own emotional reactions (as illustrated above)? Is she sensitive to the emotional reactions of others? How was Joe feeling when he entered the theatre environment, and might his behaviour have been bravado? Did Geeta take the initiative to discuss the situation with Joe directly after the incident and perhaps explain the rationale behind her intervention in terms of patient safety? Or, by waiting, was she hoping that Joe might 'know his place' and that she could reassume the status of 'senior student' as she had 'protected the patient from infection risk'? Geeta would need to review how she could have taken responsibility for acknowledging her own feelings and to what extent her autobiography had been instrumental in her behaviour. She might have acknowledged that she felt her position of trust by the theatre staff was threatened by Joe, and led to her reaction of telling Joe about the negative views of some staff, thus escalating the situation. Was she conscious of how the situation could have made Joe feel? Geeta might need to read about exercising emotional intelligence to inform her practice.

Another element of Geeta's reflection could be the way she deals with unexpected situations. As a final-year student, one could expect Geeta to be more resilient and not to be so upset by a confrontation that she needs a break. She had taken her responsibility and had acted in accordance with the NMC's Code (NMC, 2018b). You could conclude from her reaction to Joe confronting her that there had been a personal element to her response to the situation in theatre, hence her feeling personally attacked and not being able to rise above Joe's emotions and defuse the situation, using the communications skills she will have learned throughout the nursing programme.

A final point of reflection for Geeta could be around the culture in the theatre suite – a culture where registered staff are conscious of disliking a student but not taking the responsibility to discuss it with the student involved. Rather, they choose to pass the responsibility to another student without, apparently, clarifying roles, status and responsibilities. What could this say about the safety and openness of the learning environment? What does this mean in terms of labelling a student negatively? Do you think that Joe will be given a fair chance of succeeding on his placement? Could Geeta have, subconsciously, recognised this and have wanted to stay on the good side of the theatre staff?

Activity 6.4 Reflection (page 115)

Charmaine's presence helped Jerry to focus on the quality of his explanation for the benefit of Charmaine and the patient. He was also re-examining his knowledge base in the light of Charmaine's questions. Charmaine was reviewing her present knowledge to identify what adjustments she needed to make for applying it in this new care context. She was influenced by Jerry's communication style, which she viewed as a positive role model for practice.

Further reading

Cassidy, S (2009) Interpretation of competence in student assessment. *Nursing Standard*, 23(18): 39–46.

This article will help you to understand how practice supervisors use reflexivity in coming to assessment decisions and how important reflexivity is in developing competence as a nurse.

Goleman, D (2004) *Emotional Intelligence and Working with Emotional Intelligence* (omnibus). London: Bloomsbury.

This book will help you to understand the relationship between emotions and cognition, and the importance of working with emotional intelligence when dealing with people.

Hurley, J and Linsley, P (2012) *Emotional Intelligence in Health and Social Care.* London: Radcliffe.

This book will help you understand why and how to apply emotional intelligence in health- and social care situations.

Sully, P and Dallas, J (2010) *Essential Communication Skills for Nursing and Midwifery*, 2nd edn. Edinburgh: Elsevier Mosby.

This book helps to identify how you can develop appropriate communication skills for therapeutic and professional purposes.

Reflective Practice (journal)

This journal offers a variety of articles on different aspects of reflecting and practising reflexively.

Chapter 7　The reflective practitioner

Chapter aims

After reading this chapter you will be able to:

- define and identify morally active practice;
- recognise the fallibility of professional knowledge and developing practice;

(Continued)

(Continued)

- develop some strategies to manage knowledge deficits, near misses and mistakes in your practice;
- understand the need for reflecting on the complexity of decisions and consequences.

Introduction

Scenario 7.1: Debbie experiences a reflective practitioner in action

Debbie was in the third year of her nurse preparation programme. She was on a specialist placement with the *multiple sclerosis* (MS) nurse, Gill. Debbie was very interested in seeing how Gill worked with a caseload of her own patients, referring them to other health professionals as appropriate. This was a different view of nursing and one with which Debbie was not familiar. She thought about what she had observed from seeing Gill working with a variety of patients with differing degrees of illness severity. Debbie was surprised that, at times, Gill acknowledged to patients that she was not sure what was causing their symptoms, but that working together they would be able to devise an appropriate plan. When Debbie asked about this, Gill highlighted that patients were the experts in terms of what they were experiencing and their coping strategies, and explained that MS is such a variable illness, with more being discovered about it all the time.

Gill related the example of *benign MS*, which had been assumed not to cause significant nerve damage, and therefore patients developed milder symptoms that were usually non-progressive and often not taken seriously. However, recent research findings had suggested that far more significant damage was sustained within the first attack and could lie dormant until further illness and ageing activated damaged areas and potentially triggered progression. Gill used this example to explain to Debbie how important it was for the health practitioner to work with patients and constantly review their own assumptions of what was happening and what they were noticing. She also explained how it was most important to reflect on what they were doing and the aesthetics present within their practice.

Debbie realised that what she was experiencing was a reflective practitioner in action who was not afraid to acknowledge uncertainty, but who embraced it by reflecting with patients in a skilful way that drew out what concerned them the most and worked imaginatively with possibilities. Supporting this was Gill's up-to-date knowledge base, caring and concern for her patients, and her ability to interpret and review complex issues. Debbie realised Gill was the type of role model practitioner she aspired to emulate.

The example above demonstrates the changing nature of knowledge, and why it's important to reflect on practice to be able to respond effectively to change and add to the evidence base. Gill is using her knowledge of MS, but also acknowledging the unique experience of the individual, to guide the advice and support she offers. The openness to work with change in practice is a fundamental feature of the reflective practitioner. If we accept that professionals are fallible and do not always get things right, we have a point from which to start to examine the effectiveness of practice by reflecting on what might be done differently. Equally, as clients are unique human beings, they may not always respond in expected ways and such issues need to be added to the body of evidence. Being open to change and reflecting on it allows the practitioner to learn and develop. It is important for students and novice practitioners to be able to acknowledge limitations within their knowledge as well as to take ownership of potential mistakes through reflection. This will allow them to learn how to be accountable and reflective practitioners.

Activity 7.1   Reflection

Please pause for a moment to reflect on situations you may have seen in practice where, possibly retrospectively, you realise that you witnessed reflective practice. These situations could have been related to how interventions were carried out, how observations were interpreted or how communication strategies were used.

Try to answer the following questions:

- What do you remember from the situation that caused you to consider this as reflective practice?
- Did you discuss it at the time with the person involved? If you did discuss it, what did you learn from the situation? If you did not discuss it, what prevented you from doing so?

There are outline answers to these questions at the end of the chapter.

This chapter links with another book in the series, *Evidence-Based Practice in Nursing* (Ellis, 2019), and encourages students to cultivate a reflective approach to their daily experience and integrate what they are learning with their practice. We begin by examining what morally active practice is.

Morally active practice

Morally active practice is defined as critically exercising decisions based on ethical and moral principles and being able to justify these (Brechin, 2000). The morally active practitioner recognises that there are situations when some influences, such as evidence and policy, may take precedence over others, such as personal values and patient preference, which might not be reasonable. However, some ethical principles (such as equity) must be applied, so practitioners need to be aware of the consequences of their actions (Howatson-Jones, 2015a).

Our moral thinking is influenced by the cultures we have experienced and our own histories. Moral practice is informed by professional expectation, acceptability and concern for human beings, with regard to the individual in that situation at that time.

It is important to be clear about our motives and the expected consequences of our actions, as well as being respectful about people's concerns and well-being. For example, you might have strong views about people smoking when they know it is harmful. This might translate into differing attitudes towards those presenting for treatment. Even if this is repressed, it may nevertheless still be active within your thinking and, therefore, reflecting. A more extreme example might be when faced with caring for someone who is an abuser, or a person who has inflicted some harm on themselves or others. Equity means that care should be provided immaterial of personal feelings or prejudices. However, reflecting on reactions to such situations is an important part of being able to deal with them, and of learning from the experience. Consider Scenario 7.2 and then answer the questions at the end.

Scenario 7.2: Greg's morally active care

Greg was a newly qualified nurse working on a busy medical ward during his preceptorship period. Many of the patients had complex health problems and Greg often left the ward feeling exhausted with the pace of work. Greg was particularly troubled about Gina, a 26-year-old patient with diabetes. Gina had been admitted to the ward twice in the last six weeks due to binge drinking, which had affected her diabetes. Greg was strictly teetotal and found it difficult to understand why Gina was putting her health at risk in this way. Nevertheless, he set aside his background influences and tried to see things from Gina's perspective by conversing with her whenever he was undertaking nursing tasks. Greg's preceptor Ivan (who was aware he was teetotal) commented on this when they met to complete some of Greg's documentation.

Greg said he did sometimes feel uncomfortable around Gina because of her lifestyle, but through conversing with her he had developed some understanding of the reasons for her behaviour. He considered Gina's hospital admissions to be avoidable, but thought counselling might provide a route to help Gina develop coping strategies. Ivan explained what he had observed about Greg's communication style with Gina and asked Greg to write a reflective log about this situation to share at their next meeting. Ivan thought this might provide a useful start to a practice teaching session for student nurses.

Activity 7.2   Critical thinking

- What is the NMC's Code (2018b) likely to have emphasised about this situation?
- What might Greg have focused on in his reflection?
- What changes might Greg be thinking of making?

There are outline answers to these questions at the end of the chapter.

The morally active practitioner utilises a reflective rather than a judgemental approach to examine the outcomes of their actions and decisions. This means using your whole self when thinking about practice, engaging feelings and being aware of intentions.

Activity 7.3   Reflection

Use the following questions to spend a little time reflecting on your own values and beliefs.

- What is important to you and why?
- What do you find difficult to cope with and why?
- Have the answers to the above questions changed during the course of your life and, if so, why?
- How have these issues related to your practice?

There is an outline answer to this activity at the end of the chapter.

Professional experience is helpful for providing the skills necessary to develop, but it is also important to consider what we think about being a professional and how we interpret professionalism. For example, the fact that practitioners are able to negotiate the nursing environment freely, whereas patients and clients are not, puts you, as the practitioner, in a position of power. This needs to be considered with regard to how you approach your practice. Employing an authoritarian approach that places you firmly in control means that you may be cut off from learning other points of view, which also inform practice and are useful for reflecting on. Equally, when you are just following instructions and policies you may appear to be professional, but if you omit reflection on your practice all you are doing is conforming to established behaviours. This is not the same as reflecting to ensure the effectiveness and development of practice. Besides, policies and guidelines might seem to suggest that there is only one way of doing things, but we know that nursing is dynamic and changing, and that there are few things in life that are more unpredictable than people. Scenario 7.3 will help illustrate this point.

Scenario 7.3: Pavlina's professional experience

Pavlina was in the final year of her nursing programme working in a radiology department. Everything was new to her and she was worried about the radiation involved in imaging procedures. Her practice supervisor, Gabriel, asked her to read the radiation protection guidelines in her first week. Pavlina reflected after reading these. She thought about how she had felt on her first day and wondered whether patients might have similar feelings and concerns about radiation. She considered the new knowledge she had gained from reading the guidelines and how this could inform her practice.

Pavlina observed a variety of diagnostic and interventional procedures, always making sure that she was in position to reassure the patient. As the placement continued, she felt more confident to inform patients about what was happening. Gabriel involved her in setting up procedures and undertaking nursing observations. Pavlina also learned a lot during patient handovers to ward staff after procedures. She was, however, concerned that these handovers took place in a public space.

Pavlina reflected with Gabriel at the end of her placement. Gabriel told her how impressed he was with the way she had translated her reading of the radiation protection guidelines into reassuring explanations for patients. He also praised Pavlina's hard work and dedication to her learning. Pavlina told Gabriel how much she had enjoyed the variety of learning opportunities available in this placement, but she also voiced concern about patient handovers occurring in public spaces, and the way that the radiologists explained the procedure in the room and then asked the patient for their consent. Pavlina felt that this could be perceived as coercive because everyone was ready for the procedure to start. Gabriel reflected with Pavlina on these issues.

Activity 7.4   Reflection

- What do you think Pavlina has learned about professionalism in this scenario?
- What else might she have learned about effective practice through reflection with Gabriel?
- What options for change might they have considered?

There are outline answers to these questions at the end of the chapter.

When reading Scenario 7.3 you may have immediately had some further questions and thoughts about what was happening. It is for this reason that Abrandt Dahlgren et al. (2004, p15) urge practitioners to reflect 'about' practice as well as 'on' or 'in' practice. Practical awareness can develop only when such reflective thinking occurs and helps nursing as a profession to move forward. Taking responsibility for your own learning through reflecting about the practice in which you are involved is an important part of this process. We proceed now to examine how professionals might sometimes be fallible, and the role of reflection in managing this situation.

Practitioner fallibility and reflection

As a healthcare practitioner you are subjected to scrutiny from a number of directions. The NMC (2018a) sets the standards for practice and regulates professional behaviour. The government legislates the policies with which healthcare is expected to comply (Department of Health [DH], 2009, 2015), and the Quality Assurance Agency (QAA, 2014), through the Code for Higher Education, inspects the validity of teaching and assessment. With so many dictates for practice, it is hardly surprising that professionals sometimes get things wrong. Human error theory asserts that error is inevitable at some stage, but it is important to establish the reasons for flaws in judgement in order to address any problems (Armitage, 2009). Activity 7.5 will help you identify some issues that play a part in potential practitioner fallibility and, with this knowledge, to reflect on how you might avoid these issues.

Activity 7.5   Reflection

Think of a decision you made that you considered a bad decision. Try to think of what might have interfered with your ability to make judgements and decisions by considering the following questions:

- What were the circumstances?
- What was the result?
- What do you think contributed to it being a bad decision?
- What did you do afterwards?
- What do you think about it now?

Using your previous answers, now consider how to make good decisions.

As this activity is based on your own experiences there are limited answers at the end of the chapter.

The decisions that professionals make usually require them to process information and use some level of intuition and cognitive aspects (Muir, 2004). Information processing refers to making sense of all the information available in terms of what is seen, heard, felt, smelt and read (Howatson-Jones, 2015b). Intuition refers to knowledge from experience being activated by the situation and inducing a response. Cognitive aspects relate to thinking about all of this and coming to a decision. During the process of deciding, choices are analysed in terms of their possible consequences – in other words we make a risk assessment, although sometimes we might not be wholly aware of this.

Social judgement theory suggests that the problem and informational cues link to the situation on which judgements are based. The ordering of cues, according to how we perceive their importance, determines how accurate the judgement is for the actual situation (Thompson and Dowding, 2002). Creativity through remaining flexible and responsive, using information-processing skills to understand emerging data, being clear about what you are aiming for, seeking guidance as appropriate, and knowing the extent and limits of your knowledge are all contributing factors to good decision-making (Bohinc and Gradisar, 2003). This chapter links with another book in the series, *Clinical Judgement and Decision Making in Nursing* (Standing, 2017), and you are encouraged to look at this topic in more detail. However, by reading Scenario 7.4 and answering the questions at the end you may be able to identify some issues relating to practitioner fallibility.

Scenario 7.4: Elsie's escapade

Rose was in the first year of her mental health nursing programme, and working on a ward caring for older people with a cognitive impairment. One of the patients, Elsie, was quite confused. On this particular day, Elsie was found to be missing from the ward and Rose joined her practice supervisor, Mary, in searching for her. Elsie was eventually found by the main road sitting on the grass. Rose and Mary collected Elsie, putting her in a wheelchair and returning her to the ward. As Elsie was cold, Rose helped her into bed to warm up. Mary asked Rose to complete a set of observations of Elsie's temperature, pulse and blood pressure, to check on her and to include in the clinical incident form. Rose recorded these and noted that Elsie's temperature was a little low, but nothing else appeared abnormal. The doctor was also informed of Elsie's escapade, but as she appeared not to have suffered any effects he told Mary to just continue to keep an eye on her. The rest of the day was uneventful, although Elsie was restless and would call out every so often. She eventually went to sleep that night.

Rose was on the early shift the next morning. As soon as she came on duty she heard Elsie wailing. When she asked what the problem was, Mary told her that Elsie had woken up in pain. When the staff pulled her covers back they noticed that her left leg was externally rotated and shortened, a classic symptom of a fractured neck of femur. As Elsie had not been out of bed overnight (she had a urinary catheter) no one had noticed this deformity until Elsie woke in pain. Rose asked Mary how it was possible they had missed this.

Elderly bones are more fragile than younger ones because mineral density decreases with age, so even a relatively minor fall can lead to a fracture. Sometimes the muscles that encircle the hip go into rigid spasm and this can, temporarily, hold the hip in reasonable alignment. When the body relaxes, as happens in sleep, the muscles no longer maintain their hold and the deformity becomes apparent. It is unlikely that Elsie would have been able to walk on this leg, but as she returned to the ward by wheelchair this was not obvious.

Activity 7.6   Reflection

- What contributed to practitioner fallibility in this scenario?
- What should or could have been done differently?
- What might be learned from this situation?

There are outline answers to these questions at the end of the chapter.

Although the registered practitioner is accountable for their actions and the actions of those whom they are supervising, the student is responsible for ensuring that they notify changes or deficits of which they have become aware. Reflection itself may be fallible when based on inaccurate perceptions. Schön (1987) makes the point that, when understanding is not grounded in proper practice through careful examination and checking of knowing, inaccurate ideas about practice may perpetuate because the reflection itself is flawed. Reflecting with others, as discussed in Chapter 8, and analytical approaches, such as those explored in Chapter 11, can help to combat such fallibility. We proceed now to consider how to manage near misses and mistakes.

Managing deficits and near misses or mistakes

Fragmented inter-nurse and interprofessional relations can make managing deficits difficult and lead to lack of communication between groups, creating working processes that are conducive to errors. Equally, anxiety can hold back progress because a person finds it difficult to make a decision for fear of getting it wrong, and therefore relies on being told what to do by others. Without the confidence and knowledge to interrogate your practice, and that of others, poor practice and mistakes may be perpetuated as the following case study illustrates.

Case study: Rhian's experience of poor practice

Rhian was in the first year of her nursing programme and on placement in a nursing home. She was keen to make a good impression and anxious to do things correctly. A number of the patients had continence problems but, during the day, through careful observation and trips to the toilet, the problem was dealt with in a dignified way. But Rhian had started to notice, when she was on an early shift, that some of these patients had many incontinence pads in their beds, and that these were making their skin sweat and consequently the pads were sticking to them. When Rhian mentioned this to a care assistant, the care assistant told her not to interfere because this was the way things were done on the night shift. Rhian was not sure about this but did not want to make a fuss and show herself up. She decided to talk to her practice supervisor about it. When Rhian spoke to her practice supervisor, Dave, he said that it was different at night because the patients could not get up as easily to go to the toilet and so the pads were necessary. Rhian relayed that there seemed to be rather a lot of them and they were always very wet. Dave said he would look into it. However, the weeks passed, and Rhian did not see any change. She feared that perhaps she had been wrong to think this was not right. Rhian left her placement with the view that using a lot of incontinence pads at night was normal practice. Three months later, when reflecting after another placement, she realised that what she had seen in the first placement was wrong. She decided that, if she was concerned about practice again, she would challenge the practice and talk to her practice supervisor, but she would also follow it up with a link tutor.

The case study has illustrated that, without reflection, practice and developing knowledge can be difficult. The Francis (2013) report highlighted the consequences of not following through on concerns about practice. Completing Activity 7.7 explores what you might do in a similar situation.

Activity 7.7   Critical thinking

You are encouraged to look at your university and placement institution policies for raising concerns and then think about the following questions:

1.   What factors would help you recognise a concern?
2.   What might be barriers to raising a concern and how might you overcome them?
3.   How could you consolidate your learning from thinking about these processes?

As this activity is based on your experiences there is a limited answer at the end of the chapter.

Similar to Rhian in the case study, you might have recognised a concern by the uneasy feelings with which you were left. However, this is not concrete evidence and reflecting on the situation and analysing surrounding factors (as we did in Chapter 4 with the different reflective models) can help you to develop a better evidence base. Developing reflective ability is a transitional process that involves struggle, accepting the challenge, making connections, learning to reflect more deeply and sharing with others (Glaze, 2001). Rhian could have progressed from her struggle with understanding, to accepting the challenge to find out more for herself. This might, in turn, have helped her make different connections and learn. We all recognise Rhian's difficulty and challenge of questioning practice as a student. However, with practice, this does become easier – communication is, after all, a skill and combined with emotional intelligence will stand you in good stead for the rest of your career. It is, therefore, important to start learning to 'experiment' with raising concerns and 'challenging' in a skilful and professional way as early as possible. It might be of some 'comfort' to you to realise that the NMC's Code (NMC, 2018b) does attempt to support staff who raise concerns because managers are bound by the section *Preserve safety: Act without delay if you believe that there is a risk to patient safety or public protection* (items 16.4, 16.5 and 16.6). It is fortunate that Rhian was able to see 'normal' practice on her subsequent placements. Not challenging what you consider to be inferior practice because you fear recriminations will be difficult behaviour to change as a student, but also as a qualified staff member, if you do not learn the necessary skills and communication strategies. Challenging inferior practice is an important element of the NMC's Code (NMC, 2018b); please read the section *Preserve safety* (items 16.1, 16.3 and 17.1–17.3).

Mistakes can be a 'shocking' form of learning through their abrupt nature. Similarly, witnessing inferior practice can also be 'shocking' because it is unexpected and contrary to any ethical perspectives on non-maleficence, justice and equity, and the antithesis of the nursing values of care and compassion. Mistakes and inferior practice can both trigger an emotional response. Mistakes can leave you feeling emotionally upset and lower your self-esteem, and witnessing inferior practice can leave you feeling helpless and experiencing an ethical dilemma unless the situation can be resolved. By transforming the situation into learning through reflection, it will help you to regain your self-confidence. This involves considering how action, or inaction, contributed to the error, thinking about the nature of the mistake and what it means to be a professional. Responses can be categorised as emotional, cognitive and behavioural as follows.

Emotional response

Stage 1   shock and grief;

Stage 2   defending by projecting blame.

Cognitive response

Stage 3   scrutinising own practice, acknowledging shortcomings;

Stage 4   scrutinising others' contributing practice to identify influences;

Stage 5   identifying the core problem and accepting responsibility;

Stage 6   checking core knowledge.

Behavioural response

Stage 7   reflecting on the error and behaviour and how to change;

Stage 8   identifying how to improve and regain confidence.

It is important that emotional responses to difficult practice and errors are acknowledged at the start, if you are to move forward to thinking about what needs to change. Please consider Scenario 7.5.

Scenario 7.5: Roger's near miss

Roger was in the final year of his nursing programme working on a day surgery unit. The pace of work at the start of the day was quite fast, with many people arriving and needing to be prepared for theatre. Often, premedications were required and had to be given quickly. One of the patients had been ready for a while and Roger and his practice supervisor, Sarah, went to get his premedication. They checked that it was prescribed and properly signed for by the doctor, that it had not already been given and that the patient had no allergies to the drug. They then checked the patient's name band and told him that the tablets they were giving him were his premedication. The patient's wife said that he had just been given tablets in the last ten minutes. When Sarah checked with the other staff she discovered that the patient had been given his premed previously, but that the nurse had forgotten to sign for it because she was busy. Due to the alertness of the patient's wife this had been a near miss. Sarah and Roger completed a critical incident form for this episode. Sarah reported the incident to the unit manager.

During a lull later in the morning Sarah and Roger reflected on this incident. They both felt quite shaken at the near miss and angry with the nurse who had not signed after giving the premedication. Roger discussed the merits of, in future, asking patients whether they had been given the premedication already, but Sarah pointed out that patients may not know what type of drugs they had already been given. Sarah highlighted that all professionals are fallible and that the only guard against this was to follow drug administration guidelines and to learn from such incidents. What they had both learned was to ensure that documentation was completed in a timely manner and to delegate tasks that might prevent this. After this event Roger was very careful when checking any medication and also with his documentation.

Activity 7.8   Reflection

- What learning did Roger take from this incident?
- In what ways are emotional, cognitive and behavioural responses evident in Sarah's and Roger's reflections?
- If you are an experienced practitioner how might the unit manager have dealt with this incident and the nurses involved?

There are outline answers to these questions at the end of the chapter.

Regaining confidence after a mistake requires support as well as guidance in order to be ready to identify where the point of departure from effective decision-making comes. We proceed now to consider reflecting on complex decisions in order to assist with the process of identifying effectiveness.

Reflecting on complex decisions

Practice experiences incorporate perceptions and interpretations that require acting upon. The decisions you make may be simple or more complex, and you are likely to use a variety of data to come to a judgement. Subjective experience relates to how a person experiences their situation and is usually relayed through description. Interpretation may add further subjective data. An objective view, on the other hand, makes use of data that can be measured and recorded, such as vital signs and test results (Hinchliff et al., 2008). Within clinical practice, both of these views are relevant and indeed valuable.

Reflection, however, adds the possibility of looking for threads of meaning running through, and possibly between, the information produced from these approaches. Analysing these threads of meaning as additional processes helps to identify issues such as power, including lack of it, and how these relate to the situation. The meaning of the analysis is not always immediately obvious, and reflection endeavours to draw this out in order to read situations more accurately, to develop personal decision-making, and to improve or maintain the efficiency and effectiveness of practice. Reading Scenario 7.6 and thinking about the question at the end will help you understand these processes further.

Scenario 7.6: Natasha's experience of under-age consent

Natasha was near the end of the second year of her nursing programme and working in an A&E unit. On this particular shift, a 15-year-old girl – Milly – was brought in

(Continued)

(Continued)

with a suspected ectopic pregnancy. Milly was adamant that she did not want her mother to know. Natasha recorded her vital signs of temperature, pulse, respirations and blood pressure, and noted that Milly's pulse was raised and her blood pressure was lower than normal. Natasha started to develop a conversation with Milly while she undertook this task and asked her why she did not want her mother to know. Milly told Natasha that she had always felt judged by her mother, who did not like her friends and was always criticising her. The situation she was now in would only confirm to her mother that she was 'no good', as she put it. Milly said that she mostly stayed with friends and spent as little time at home as possible. Milly asked Natasha to call her boyfriend instead.

After Milly had had an ultrasound scan, the obstetrician and gynaecological surgeon decided that she would need an operation. Milly was still adamant that she did not want her mother to know. Her boyfriend was not interested in staying, saying he would 'see her later'. Milly went to theatre without her mother knowing and with Natasha accompanying her. Natasha, only four years older, wondered about the sense of this.

Activity 7.9   Reflection

- What are the main issues within this scenario?
- Who holds the power and in what way?
- What alternatives were available to the practitioners concerned?

There are outline answers to these questions at the end of the chapter.

Chapter summary

This chapter has illustrated a number of ways in which you can develop as a reflective practitioner. Through the examples and scenarios, it has highlighted the importance of learning from mistakes and has offered opportunities for learning to challenge poor practice in ourselves and in others. By continuing to use reflection to inform your practice, you will be able to recognise the connections between events and how you are progressing, as well as how issues such as power are important to the outcome of decisions. The importance of sharing your reflections in order to develop practice within the wider profession of nursing is continued in Chapter 8, which looks at forms of reflecting with others.

Activities and scenarios: Brief outline answers

Activity 7.1 Reflection (page 121)

You may have observed someone interacting with a service user or family member that triggered your attention. For example, this could have been the way in which an intimate closeness was established in the midst of a busy environment, or it could have been how a potentially escalating situation was defused. Was it something in the person's body language, tone of voice, eye contact or choice of words that you noticed? It would be interesting to find out to what degree the person was consciously choosing to exercise these strategies or whether this was a way of being. Carper (1978) would describe this as an aesthetic pattern of knowing. You might find it interesting to read more on this topic as numerous authors make the link of reflective practice, comfort, caring and compassion (another of the 6 Cs), for example, Hawley (2000), Nåden and Eriksson (2004), Wiman and Wikblad (2004), Nåden and Sæteren (2006) and Nilsson et al. (2008).

It is also interesting to ponder on whether you did or did not discuss this with the person at the time and your rationale behind this decision. In hindsight, do you possibly think that you may have missed an opportunity to learn from a good example that someone was (unconsciously) providing?

Activity 7.2 Critical thinking on Greg's morally active care (page 123)

The NMC's Code (NMC, 2018b) makes it clear that practitioners should avoid making assumptions (please see the sections *Promote professionalism and trust* [items 20.3, 20.5 and 20.7] and *Prioritise people* [items 1.1, 1.3 and 1.5]). Taking these aspects of the Code into account, Greg might have reflected on how his background was influencing his prejudices about Gina. Depending on his knowledge base, he could have explored potential reasons for her drinking and methods of coping with her diabetes, and how this fits with information he has gained from talking with Gina. In addition, Greg might be thinking of how he can develop his attitude and communication style to be more compassionate. It is likely that Greg would want to discuss ideas about this with Ivan at their next meeting, to help him develop a personal learning/action plan for himself to work on these aspects of his professional development, but Greg could also ask Ivan to work with him to develop a practice learning session for students on the ward.

Activity 7.3 Reflection (page 123)

You might have identified that honesty from yourself and others is important to you so that both parties can be relied on. You may also have found that doing as you would be done by is a central value for you, so that you can be trusted. You might also have identified that you find unkindness difficult to witness because of the emotional distress it can cause. It is likely you will have become aware of changes in your values and beliefs when entering your teenage years and when embarking on working life, and possibly parenthood. You might even have noticed changes when entering your nursing programme. Changes are likely to have resulted from life experience modifying and altering value responses, although core values will remain. These issues might relate to your practice, in how you think about team working, and your attitudes to patients, siblings, friends and colleagues.

It is important to be mindful of changes and how they affect you, your behaviour and your reactions to events and situations. Remember that the things that you see or will have seen in the first year of nursing most people do not experience in their entire lives. It is inevitable that we change through our experiences and we should remember to include those who are important to us in this change, otherwise we risk losing people along the way and perhaps even ourselves, as discussed in Chapter 6 in relation to emotional labour.

Activity 7.4 Reflection on Pavlina's professional experience (page 124)

Pavlina will have learned that different professionals can work as a team and the importance of policy and guidelines for informing practice. Her reflection with Gabriel highlighted that she can translate her knowledge into explanations to reassure patients. During their reflection they might consider the power relationships between different staff groups. They might also consider whether consent was really informed when taken just before the procedure. The options for change that they might have thought about could include:

- The radiologists could visit inpatients on wards, give explanations and obtain consent in the morning. Attendance of outpatients for appointments can imply consent, but obtaining final consent and answering questions could be done in private.
- Handover to ward staff could be undertaken in an office with observations and wound site checks undertaken in a procedure room.

Pavlina is likely to have left this placement with a view of professionalism that is open to feedback and constantly evolving to develop practice. However, a point of reflection would be why Pavlina waited until the end of her placement to raise the issue of privacy and confidentiality. This could have been discussed while she was still in the placement area, so that she had the opportunity to help implement the change. The final year of the programme is the most opportune moment to practise leadership and initiate change.

Activity 7.5 Reflection (page 125)

Contributing factors impacting on your decision-making may range from tiredness and overwork to stress and lack of knowledge. Equally, not taking account of the patient's view may mean that interventions fail due to non-adherence. You are likely to have tried to rectify the decision and rebuild your self-esteem. However, without reflecting on the quality of the decision and the surrounding circumstances, not all the deficits might have been noticed, so only a partial solution may have been put in place. With regard to tiredness and stress, please refer to the NMC's Code (NMC, 2018b), item 2.10, which states the expectation that nurses need to maintain an appropriate level of health.

Reflection helps to rebuild confidence and self-esteem so, if you have not reflected, you might view the decision with shame and doubt yourself. When considering how to make good decisions in response to your reflection, you might identify that including others in the decision-making processes could help to overcome stress and lack of knowledge. Equally, including the patient could also help avoid non-adherence. Certainly, including the patient in decision-making processes is in keeping with the NMC's Code (NMC, 2018b); please consider *Prioritise people* (items 2.1–2.6).

Activity 7.6 Reflection on Elsie's escapade (page 127)

The assumption was that Elsie's behaviour was related solely to her confusion and, as her observations were normal, there was nothing wrong. It is easy to dismiss possible cues in such a way and the situation should have been reviewed critically. This would have entailed asking questions, such as:

- What might have contributed to Elsie ending up sitting on the grass?
- Is the way she is calling different from usual?
- What is triggering it?
- What calms her?

Nobody witnessed how Elsie ended up sitting on the grass, so a thorough physical examination should have been carried out. This might have alerted nurses to more signs, which would have given a reason for the doctor to see Elsie. Other measurements, such as oxygen saturation and blood sugar, might have been appropriate to ascertain why she had ended up sitting. It is likely the nurses will have had to review and justify their decision-making process via a patient safety incident form and provide statements. Students involved in such situations would also be required to provide written testaments.

The learning from this situation could be the need for assertive decision-making and leadership that read the cues from situations accurately. Continual assessment focusing on the patient, and not relying only on monitoring devices, is an essential part of this process. Recognising that a situation has changed comes from experience, but also through being open-minded and having a reflective attitude that does not accept circumstances at face value. This is challenging on long stay or residential units with a low turnover of clients and where service users are generally stable. It is human to assume that small changes in behaviour are just part of who the person is, and this is often the case, but we need to be mindful that service users are, in fact, strangers to us and we need to remember that we do not know all their idiosyncrasies. We should be mindful that this situation potentially breaches the NMC's Code (NMC, 2018b). Please consider which sections of the Code are appropriate. For example, you might want to look at *Practise effectively* (items 10.1–10.4) and *Preserve safety* (items 14.1–14.3, 19.1 and 19.2).

Activity 7.7 Critical thinking (page 128)

Some factors that might cause concern are:

- feeling uneasy;
- seeing actions and behaviours that are contrary to what you have been taught;
- seeing negative effects for patients;
- inaction by staff to address issues.

Barriers to raising concerns might be:

- not wanting to draw attention to yourself;
- not being sure of your evidence;
- not knowing the process to follow.

Consolidating your learning might involve reflecting on your experience and writing a critically reflective account (please see Chapter 11 for more information).

Activity 7.8 Reflection on Roger's near miss (page 131)

Roger learned that mistakes can still happen, even with the correct checking procedures, when there have been earlier errors in a chain of events. He has learned to ensure that his documentation is carried out in a timely manner and the importance of delegation when the unit is busy.

Sarah and Roger both responded emotionally to the near miss, with anger aimed at the colleague who had not documented correctly. Thinking about the incident they considered their options, although Roger's suggestion of asking the patient is not entirely reliable and could send a message that staff might be incompetent. Sarah and Roger's responses were to ensure timely documentation when involved in drug administration.

The unit manager should undertake group reflection with the staff concerned, and develop this into refresher training for all staff to prevent such an incident happening again. Taking an educative rather than a punitive approach, the unit manager is likely to enable the staff to regain self-esteem and develop good practice. Another option would be regular clinical supervision for staff to help them reflect on practice in a confidential environment.

Please read the appropriate sections of the NMC's Code (NMC, 2018b), for example, *Preserve safety* (items 14.1–14.3, 18.2–18.4, 19.1 and 19.2).

Activity 7.9 Reflection on Natasha's experience of under-age consent (page 132)

The main issues are Milly's serious clinical condition, her request for confidentiality, Milly's age, her mental competence and the rights of her mother. The clinical danger due to a possible ectopic rupture can cause major haemorrhage, and requires immediate surgery. Since the Gillick Law in 1985 (National Society for the Prevention of Cruelty to Children or NSPCC, 2018), doctors are required to assess the competency of minors to make their own decisions. If Milly is deemed competent and fully understands the facts of the situation, she may be considered competent to make the decision and give consent. However, it is for the doctor to decide whether the complexity of the decision is in keeping with the limits of consent and Milly's competence. A further challenge is an ethical dilemma between respecting patient confidentiality and safeguarding an under-age person.

Other alternatives might have been to persuade Milly to tell her mother, or to allow a member of the team to do so, or to inform another member of the family to whom she felt able to talk. Natasha should be mindful not to superimpose her subjective experience on to that of Milly. The objective data of the vital signs recording and the ultrasound have identified the clinical urgency, and Milly's subjective experience has informed her decision.

As indicated, this is a difficult situation, so please consult the NMC's Code (NMC, 2018b), *Prioritise people* (items 1.1, 1.3, 1.5, 5.1, 5.2, 5.4 and 5.5) and *Practise effectively* (items 6.1 and 10.1–10.5).

For further reading on ethical decision-making, please see another book in the series: *Understanding Ethics for Nursing Students* (Ellis, 2017).

Further reading

Howatson-Jones, L, Standing, M and Roberts, S (2015) *Patient Assessment and Care Planning in Nursing*, 2nd edn. London: Sage.

This book looks at different issues relating to the assessment and care of patients. It will help you understand and deal with some of the dilemmas that can arise in practice, and the role of reflection in helping to make your decisions.

Johns, C (ed.) (2013) *Becoming a Reflective Practitioner*, 4th edn. Chichester: John Wiley & Sons, Inc.

This book will help you to gain an understanding of developing as a reflective practitioner in different contexts and through creative means.

Standing, M (2017) *Clinical Judgement and Decision-Making for Nursing Students*, 3rd edn. London: Sage.

This book offers a matrix model for decision-making illustrated by case studies.

Useful websites

Nursing and Midwifery Council Fitness for Practise hearing outcomes: **www.nmc-uk.org/hearings**

Click on the hearing you want to look at and then on the outcomes for the detail of the case. Reading cases from the NMC's website will help you to comprehend the significance of justifying your practice and the importance of continuing to reflect on it in order to ensure your effectiveness.

International Practice Development Journal: **www.fons.org/library/journal.aspx**

This is a free access international journal that publishes articles relating to practice development, many of which involve reflection and how to be a reflective practitioner. Type reflection in the search box to find a list of relevant volumes. You may even want to submit a reflection for potential publication yourself!

Chapter 8 Guided reflection and reflecting with others

NMC Standards of Proficiency for Registered Nurses

This chapter will address the following platforms and proficiencies:

Platform 1: Being an accountable professional

1.10 Demonstrate resilience and emotional intelligence and be capable of explaining the rationale that influences their judgements and decisions in routine, complex and challenging situations.

1.17 Take responsibility for continuous self-reflection, seeking and responding to support and feedback to develop their professional knowledge and skills.

Platform 5: Leading and managing nursing care and working in teams

5.6 Exhibit leadership potential by demonstrating an ability to guide, support and motivate individualism and interact confidently with other members of the care team.

5.10 Contribute to supervision and team reflection activities to promote improvements in practice and services.

Chapter aims

After reading this chapter you will be able to:

- identify ways of dealing with the emotional labour of caring work;
- reflect in a group as part of action learning;
- reflect with other professionals;
- define guided reflection;
- understand clinical supervision frameworks and models.

Introduction

Scenario 8.1: Sally's experience with death and dying

Sally was in the second year of her nursing programme and on a placement at a hospice. She had been very nervous about going there because she was not sure whether she would be able to cope with this type of nursing. She imagined that all the patients would be dying and that it would be a very depressing place to work in. She was surprised to find that there were a variety of patients and that there was a cheerful atmosphere. The nurses worked efficiently but made sure that they also gave a lot of time to the patients. Sharon, Sally's practice supervisor, assigned Amanda – a woman who had been treated for breast cancer but who now had lung and bone *metastases* – for Sally to look after over a number of shifts.

Sally found that she and Amanda had many things in common, even though Amanda was ten years older than her. Amanda used to be a dancer, but when she became ill the treatments exhausted her too much to continue. Sally loved salsa dancing and went out most weekends to a salsa bar with her friends. She told Amanda about some of their escapades, which made her laugh. As Amanda weakened, Sally became increasingly involved in her personal care. On Sally's last placement shift she went into Amanda's room and found her breathing had changed. Sharon told her that this was the last stage before imminent death and encouraged Sally to stay with Amanda so she would not be alone, because she had no family nearby. Sharon felt that Sally was ready for this last important care that she could offer Amanda. Sally wanted to do this. Amanda died peacefully three hours later.

Sharon came in to help Sally prepare Amanda and to give her a chance to talk about this last stage of nursing. Sally said she could understand now why nurses said they found this type of nursing satisfying. She told Sharon how privileged she felt to be there at the end, supporting Amanda through this difficult phase. As they prepared Amanda, Sharon also asked Sally to describe the changes she had witnessed in Amanda as she approached death and afterwards. Sharon's purpose for doing this was twofold. First, it would help Sally to recognise signs and stages of death and, second, it would help her to disengage from emotional attachment with Amanda so she could leave the shift composed. Through the process of preparation Sally felt that they had been respectful of Amanda and she left the shift feeling sad but also satisfied with her care.

Back at the university, Sally was kept busy with thinking about assignments and completing her course work. It was a few weeks later when Sally was sharing the practice experience with other students on her programme during a class that she realised how profoundly this experience had affected her. As the tutor helped the group to reflect on their experiences, she encouraged them to explore and analyse their responses and decisions, and what sense they were making of what was happening at the time and afterwards. Sally realised that her reaction to the situation stemmed from the emotional impact that this event had had on her. She had been close to Amanda and was sad to have that connection broken. She also felt concern about what Amanda might have been feeling at the end. Sally had made use of touch to communicate her concern and talked quietly to Amanda. Ann, one of the class members, suggested that Sally and Sharon might have been trying to control the situation, because Amanda had no way of telling them whether she wanted this type of communication or not. The tutor also asked Sally to think about how this situation might differ if she and Amanda were from markedly different cultural and social backgrounds.

Sally was struck by the fact that it was difficult to determine what patients wanted during end-of-life care, because beyond a certain point nursing was based on nurses' assumptions, intuition and experience, and not necessarily on patients' wishes. This could potentially make the experience extremely variable for the person if the nurses' assumptions were wrong. Sally thought about conversations she had overheard, talking about patients having a difficult death because they would not 'let go'. Sally wondered about the accuracy of such judgements. Sally also wondered how she would manage in different cultural situations. This was a challenging thought for Sally as she considered the possibilities of this care experience. The process of reflection had moved her from an emotional position to thinking about her own practice.

The example in Scenario 8.1 is offered to help illustrate how reflective questioning from others can add depth to reflection and develop a wider understanding. Good facilitation helps to contain the anxiety that might surround such a process. As you progress through your nursing programme and your career in healthcare, opportunities to learn from the experience of others arise. This includes interprofessional learning activities that form part of the nursing programme and when working with the multidisciplinary team in practice.

This chapter considers how guided reflection can deepen your understanding and analysis of situations, experiences and decisions, and how reflecting with others can offer support. Within this also lies a discussion of the increasing importance of skilful supervision to make sense of changing roles, and the challenges that healthcare professionals face on a daily basis. This chapter builds on the previous ones by drawing on different professional cultures and styles of guided reflection to identify how reflection, in its varying forms, is applicable across a growing range of professions, and how increased interprofessional working and learning contribute to shared reflective opportunities. The chapter identifies the spaces that exist between practitioners and how these might be facilitated to be compelling to reflective learning and personal development, in order to develop better understanding of practice.

Ways of dealing with the emotional residues of caring work

Caring work inevitably leaves some emotional imprints and can, if not monitored, result in emotional fatigue or burnout. These unresolved emotions are also known as emotional residue (Lachman, 2016). When reflecting, actions and relationships are scrutinised and critiqued, and your personal identity becomes increasingly prominent as you develop. Examining an event means that cultural, social, historical and psychological aspects are considered when giving an account (van Boven et al., 2003), for example, what led up to the event, what particular groups of people were involved, their perspectives and interpretations, and how people might be feeling. Learning can provoke anxiety and feelings of vulnerability by admitting uncertainty and being open to shift your thinking, and possibly even reframe your beliefs and values. Please undertake Activity 8.1 using the example in Scenario 8.1 to apply these ideas, in order to help develop your understanding.

Activity 8.1   Reflection

Read the example in Scenario 8.1 again. Now examine what you perceive are the main cultural, historical and psychological aspects of the situation for those involved. Are these different for the various people and, if so, how are they different? You may want to consider the people involved in the hospice and university settings. Now imagine yourself in Sally's place. Are your perceptions the same or have they changed? If so, how have they changed and is there a relationship with the stage of preparation you are at?

There is an outline answer to this activity at the end of the chapter.

When undertaking Activity 8.1, you might have been challenged to confront your views and fears about nursing a dying person, and how different cultures think about dying. You might also have questioned whether you were 'up to it'. You might have thought about similar situations that might be a problem for you. Shame and embarrassment are often experienced in the workplace and may occur within supervisory relationships (Lynch et al., 2008). For example, if you get something wrong or don't know the answer to a question, you may worry that your practice supervisor thinks less of you as a person and as a nurse. Anxiety can affect your confidence and make you prone to mistakes that you would not normally make. Relationships that are supportive and secure enough to allow exploration of thoughts and feelings can provide a form of containment for anxiety (Holmes, 2005). Building a good relationship with your practice supervisor or colleagues is a joint venture and responsibility. You are encouraged to consider Scenario 8.2 and answer the questions in Activity 8.2 to help you think about this.

Scenario 8.2: Veronica's first day on a new placement

Veronica was in the first year of her mental health nursing programme, and today was the first day of her placement with the community mental health nurses. She was excited about this placement because she thought the community might be a place where she would like to work in the future. She met Greg, her practice supervisor, at the community nurses' base. Greg welcomed Veronica and introduced her to other members of the team. He explained who people were and how things worked. He also filled her in on what they would be doing that day. Their first visit was to see Harry, a 65-year-old man who lived alone. Veronica was taken aback by the state of his home. There were newspapers piled up everywhere and what appeared to be bags of rubbish. The smell was overpowering. Greg checked that Harry was taking his medication and had a chat with him and then they left. The morning continued to be busy, but at lunchtime Greg sat down with Veronica and asked her if she was all right because he had picked up on her reaction when they visited Harry. Veronica shared her feelings of shock that anybody would want to live like that. She asked Greg how Harry could get into such a state. Greg asked her to think about some of the ways she tried to maintain control in her own life. They then reflected on some of the potential causes of Harry's behaviour and how to support him. Veronica went home that day with a different perspective of community mental health nursing, but she also felt Greg had supported her without making her feel silly.

Activity 8.2   Reflection

- What are the main issues in this scenario?
- In what other ways could Greg further support Veronica?
- What else could Veronica do to enhance her understanding?

There are outline answers to these questions at the end of the chapter.

Scenario 8.2 will have helped you to critically review what is going on in situations that you might experience as difficult. Taking ownership of the situation and looking for solutions can be challenging. Critically examining events may also challenge your accepted identity by highlighting weaknesses of which you may not have been aware.

Supported self-awareness helps to hold the tension of confronted identity and facilitate reconstructions that lead to learning and change (Lindsay, 2006). Facilitating such learning is a key part of your practice supervisor's role, but being open to developing insight is a key part of yours. We proceed now to consider how reflecting in a group can help to develop such critical awareness and how this might be sustained through the process of action learning.

Reflecting in a group as part of action learning

Developmental journeys are made up of stories, some of which may be care stories and some of which relate to the practitioner (Bishop, 2007). Action learning is a process that reflects on real-life situations with a group of practitioners in order to develop problem solving and knowledge (Dawber, 2012). It draws together knowledge, experiential learning and creativity to come to new solutions. The importance is the spiral of continuity, which takes learning forward and transforms it into action. Group involvement is vital for achieving depth of reflection and breadth of consideration of potential solutions, and for encouragement and support. The roles of various group members are as follows.

> The *presenter* needs to be open to feedback and able to explain the action plan being taken forward at the end of the session, in order to retain ownership of the problem. The session starts with the presenter proposing an issue and presenting it in such a way that group members can understand it, so the message needs to be communicated succinctly (5–10 minutes).

> *Group members* ask questions to clarify the problem and offer reflective insights to possible surrounding factors and other ways of viewing the situation. When the group members have clarified any points that were unclear, the presenter moves to sit outside the perimeter of the group to listen and take notes. The group members then discuss the merits of potential solutions to the issue and reflect on possible consequences that might arise from these, to enable an informed choice to be made. They remain focused on the issue at hand (15–20 minutes).

Normally there would be an optional *break* (5 minutes) at this point to allow the presenter to collect their thoughts.

> The *presenter* returns to the group after the break once they have completed their deliberations. The presenter then reflects on what the group has discussed, shares what they have learned from listening to the group discussing the issue they had presented, and puts forward their thoughts and ideas for an action plan (5–10 minutes).

> The *facilitator* attends and observes the group process, adding challenge, reflective insights and support as required. If necessary, the facilitator summarises the learning and actions at key stages of the group process, to keep things on track.

Clearly, confidentiality is a founding principle of such group working; without trusting that what is discussed will be kept within the group, it will be difficult for group members to share openly. Consequently, when such groups are set up they will often start with a contracting exercise, in which the group agree on the rules for engagement and individual and group responsibilities, with confidentiality being a fundamental rule. Being a group member means giving a commitment not only to keep discussions confidential, but also to demonstrate commitment to the group through attendance and contribution to the discussions. This helps to demonstrate respect for the value of working together. Sitting things out means that the learning environment, necessary for individuals and the group to learn, is not sustained.

Scenario 8.3: Matt's experience of active learning

Matt was part of an action learning group that had been set up in partnership between the university and practice. The group met monthly to share and discuss practice and identify their learning from this process. Matt was working on a medical ward, which he was finding rather boring compared with his previous placement, which had been a clinical decisions unit that was very fast paced and busy.

At this month's action learning meeting, Matt was invited to talk about his practice. Matt spoke about a patient he had admitted with chronic pulmonary disease who had complex health and social issues, and was not co-operating with the advice he was given. Astrid, a member of the action learning group, asked Matt to re-examine the language he had used when presenting the case. Matt realised he had been talking about 'patients' rather than 'people'. At first, on hearing Astrid's comment, Matt became defensive and his response within the group seemed to mirror his attitude towards people in his care. The facilitator observed the group process and allowed them space to resolve the situation. This worked well, and the group was able to de-escalate the situation. The action learning group then discussed what effect labelling might have on the people for whom they were caring and how they responded. In addition, Matt's response was discussed and the effect this might have on his experience of the medical ward he was on, and how this could be turned around. Matt came away from this action learning session feeling that he had actively learned something about communication and that his emotional response was possibly due to his frustration with his current placement.

The purpose of group reflection is to consolidate and develop professional knowledge and practice. Active learning is something that happens when everyday practice is re-examined and where new ways of working are considered which may take you out of your comfort zone (McCormack et al., 2013). In Scenario 8.3 Matt had been asked to reconsider his everyday language about working and realised that the way he refers to people and categorises them is not person centred. This is active learning because of his recognition of how he uses language and the possibility of changing it. He also realised that he should change his passive–aggressive, disinterested attitude on the ward to being proactive and discussing his learning needs and objectives. Connections that support the learner in practice draw on ideas of the development of the 'professional craft' (Titchen et al., 2004, p108), which relates to you as a practitioner and how you engage with developing your knowledge and skills base. Support of practical and critical thinking processes are ways in which others help to facilitate your development of nursing knowledge, but it is through actively learning with others that you can consolidate this knowledge, recognising your unique contribution, and expanding the skills base and confidence in your performance. Read Scenario 8.4 on the craft of nursing to develop your understanding of what this means.

Scenario 8.4: Anita's administration of an injection

Anita is an experienced staff nurse with whom you are working, but not your practice supervisor. She has been a qualified nurse for 20 years and has worked on the unit you are on for 10 years. Today she has asked you to come and observe her administering an injection in order to develop your learning of this technique. Anita begins by starting to explain to Betty (the patient) what she has planned, and to gain her consent. Betty does not really like needles. Anita returns to the clinical room with Betty's drug chart and checks it carefully, washes her hands and starts to gather the necessary equipment together. All the while she is explaining to you what she is doing, and why, and asking you questions. She checks the drug ampoule and carefully draws up the drug with no spillage and little air being introduced into the syringe. She expels any air bubbles carefully into the vial to avoid drug spray. When you both arrive at Betty's bedside, Anita asks you to talk quietly to Betty and hold her hand while she prepares the area for injection. With swift, smooth, deft movements Anita swabs the skin, inserts the needle, injects the drug and removes the needle again, pressing slightly to stem any leakage and reassuring Betty calmly. Betty has hardly noticed the injection. This whole episode has taken less than 10 minutes.

You contrast Anita's fluidity with your own clumsy technique when administering your first injection. Skin is tougher than appears in this exemplar, so the efficiency of Anita's movements must be related to her expertise. The next time, you observe Anita much more closely in order to analyse what she is adding. You note her ease of communication, which relaxes the patient, and immediately makes the insertion of the needle easier. This first step appears crucial to the whole proceedings and makes the procedure less task oriented and more patient focused. You observe the co-ordination occurring between Anita's swabbing of the skin and insertion and withdrawal of the needle, and the attention that Anita gives to the detail of her patient's reaction and physical consequences. Patient comfort and procedural efficiency are both important.

Within Scenario 8.4 Anita has developed fluidity from undertaking the procedure many times and from the slight adjustments she has learned each time in how a patient moves, responds and perhaps even flinches. The procedure has become second nature: she does not need to think about it and is able to explain and 'do' at the same time. This illustrates that the knowledge has become embedded (Sennett, 2008). However, Anita's prime focus is not the 'task' but the person. How she communicates with the patient is implied as much in the skill she exhibits. Identifying how your practice interfaces with others is an important part of developing craft knowledge, by helping to highlight what is special to the nursing role and how others can contribute to developing this knowledge in other ways. It is very powerful to have a strong role model to whom we can aspire, but it is also easy for inexperienced practitioners to become uncertain when they compare their skills with those executed by experienced colleagues. Please be mindful that this is a normal process of development. Benner (1984) discusses this development in terms of five levels of experience and explains how we view an intervention as a number of discrete actions when we learn something new but, as we progress, we learn to see it contextually as Anita illustrated in Scenario 8.4.

So far, we have focused on learning from and with nursing colleagues. We proceed now to consider the value of reflection with other professionals.

Reflecting with other professionals

Following the Francis (2013) report, the quality agenda is focused on developing the whole workforce to provide high-quality care based on principles of quality, patient-centredness, flexibility, valuing people, clinical relevance and promoting life-long learning (Department of Health [DH], 2008). Boundaries are becoming blurred, and teaching, learning and supervision opportunities arise for the novice, as well as the expert practitioner, as roles expand. Reflection is not just about what has been learned, but also about how the professional is changing. This is of particular significance when growing as a professional and how you develop reflective questions. As roles change and new ways of thinking become apparent, the implications for you as a growing professional are also important. Reflecting with other professionals can help to put this into perspective.

Completing Activity 8.3 will help you to find ways of doing this.

Activity 8.3   Reflection

Think back to your last few practice experiences and consider where your practice interfaced with that of other professionals. Write a list of all the professions you have identified. Now consider what opportunities there might have been within these areas to share practice and develop learning.

(Continued)

(Continued)

If you are an experienced practitioner, consider also how you can develop opportunities for learning from other professionals for students and for yourself.

Now think about your university programme and list any other professionals that you learn with. Consider what opportunities there might be to share practice and develop learning.

Review your findings and draw up an action plan for how you might be able to develop or take advantage of reflecting with other professionals. Identify what your objectives for doing so might be by drafting some reflective questions.

There is an outline answer to this activity at the end of the chapter.

The answers that you might have found when undertaking this activity enable you to exert some agency in your own learning, and proactively plan how you can expand your knowledge of other professions and share practice. The interprofessional approach is important to open up possibilities and thereby enhance practice. However, for the novice this may be difficult and, where there are tensions between different professional groups, the process may be better supported by inclusion of a guide who can facilitate reflection. We proceed now to consider the role of guided reflection.

Guided reflection

Guided reflection is defined as reflection that, through the questioning and insights of another more experienced practitioner, can get beneath the surface of experience. The guide helps the practitioner to reveal self-deceptions and their limits, as well as supplying support and encouragement to deepen learning (Johns, 2010). In this way it becomes possible to peel back layers of what may initially be perceived as routine practice to reach the essence of deeper learning underneath, much as peeling back the layers of an onion intensifies the chemical effects of the aroma.

During guided reflection, the practitioner is expected to confront self-deceptions and distortions of their perceptions. Consequently, an experienced and qualified person is required, and it is important that facilitation is supportive and well thought out, and that there is mutual trust between the guide and the practitioner. Facilitating containment involves setting clear boundaries and providing structure so that people do not lose themselves in unnecessary and irrelevant detail, but remain focused on what they are supposed to be doing (Thorndycraft and McCabe, 2008). The following case study helps illustrate how guided reflection might be used to reflect on a critical incident. The aim would be to provide the support required to deal with emotional residues and to develop reflective learning.

Case study: Jameel's experience of sudden life-changing injuries

Jameel was in the third year of his nursing programme working in A&E. He was working on the late shift on a busy Saturday afternoon when the emergency phone rang with a message to say that there had been a serious accident and four children were being brought in with burns. They had been playing with cellulose thinners and matches and there had been an explosion. One child had 80 per cent burns and the other three had less, but still significant injuries. Jameel helped to prepare the resuscitation area ready for the arrival of the children. He noted that none came with parents or other adults. There was a lot of noise and confusion when their parents arrived. Jameel tried to reassure them as best he could. Jameel and his practice supervisor Ricardo accompanied one of the children called Bobby – who had significant face and chest burns – as he was transferred by ambulance to a burns unit. On their way back, Jameel asked Ricardo what the future held for Bobby. Ricardo replied that Bobby would need many operations as he grew and would also need psychological support to cope with disfigurement. Jameel left the shift feeling disturbed about a number of aspects related to this incident. He wondered why no adult had been aware of where the children were or what they were doing. He also wanted to find out more about the treatment options and potential outcomes.

The next day Ricardo met with Jameel during the morning break because he realised that Jameel had been disturbed by the incident. Ricardo explained they had 15 minutes for the meeting and explored with Jameel how he felt about the incident. Jameel said he found it difficult to understand why no adult knew where the children were or what they were doing because in his culture children were much more closely supervised. He also said he wanted to find out more about burns and their treatment because this was something with which he had little experience. Jameel and Ricardo explored differences in culture and some of the social reasons why children might play alone unsupervised. Ricardo gave Jameel some references and links on burn injuries and their treatments to follow up and made arrangements to discuss these further with him at their next review meeting. Ricardo helped Jameel to see that, although he had not been able to get very involved in the initial care of the children, he had performed a valuable task of reassuring the parents despite his concerns.

This case study has demonstrated the importance of guided reflection after critical incidents such as these, because they might result in sudden life-changing situations. However, guided reflection is equally important for reflecting on everyday practice in order to review what you do and how to improve it. Clinical supervision is a form of guided reflection that can enable you to do this. The next section explains what clinical supervision is, what it is not, and some of the models and frameworks that are used.

Clinical supervision frameworks

Clinical supervision is a practice-focused relationship with a professional that enables you to work through emotionally charged situations to release stress, and explore and reflect on your work, in order to gain constructive feedback and affirmation of effective practice (Freshwater et al., 2007). The experienced professional is the supervisor and the person reflecting is the supervisee. Clinical supervision is relevant because it connects with various forms of support and has a role within quality agendas for practice (Morton-Cooper and Palmer, 2000). Clinical supervision is a form of experiential learning that supports reflective examination of practice and planning of development (Milne, 2009).

Variations on using clinical supervision include autobiographical reports from colleagues, vignettes from supervisee and supervisor, and educational input. Networking with other disciplines to share supervisors can enrich the learning process (Howatson-Jones, 2003). These variations have relevance to the facilitation and tasks of supervision. Support and clarity of boundaries of responsibility are crucial to achieve learning and to avoid doing harm through the clinical supervision process (Phelan et al., 2006). This is important, because clinical supervision makes professionals think about their self-concept as practitioners. Careful planning of objectives and goals, working creatively through the harnessing of technology such as Skype or synchronous blogging, using existing forums such as progress meetings for the student, and ward meetings for the more experienced practitioner to provide clarification, are all ways to consider how implementation might be broadened. The managerial role in terms of actual supervision and caring for the well-being of the workforce is crucial to establishing an effective supervision programme that enables practitioners of all abilities and stages of progression to learn and feel good about themselves (van Ooijen, 2013). When considering your first qualified role or, as a qualified member of staff, one of the provisions you might want to think about is whether the organisation to which you are applying offers clinical supervision to its staff. If you are already employed, you could consider how clinical supervision could be implemented or improved.

The Nursing and Midwifery Council (NMC, 2006) identifies clinical supervision as being important and asserts the following principles:

- Clinical supervision supports practice.
- Clinical supervision is a practice-focused relationship.
- Clinical supervision should be developed according to local need and circumstances.
- Ground rules should be agreed to support openness and transparency.

- Every practitioner should have access.
- There should be preparation for supervisors.
- Evaluation of clinical supervision should take place to determine influence on care.

However, clinical supervision is only as effective as practitioners' ability to be self-aware, and have some insight into their own feelings and behaviours. Key stages of the reflective process within clinical supervision include the following.

- *Self-awareness*: the process of getting to know feelings, attitudes and values;
- *Description*: the ability to recognise and recollect key events;
- *Critical analysis*: examining components, challenging assumptions and exploring alternatives;
- *Synthesis*: integration of new knowledge and identifying action;
- *Evaluation*: making judgements about the value of the experience.

Self-awareness is about the kind of relationship you have with yourself. For example, are you critical of yourself, too demanding in your expectations or not demanding enough? Maybe there are times when your appraisal of yourself might not be accurate or realistic. For example, you might think that you know how to do something because you have completed the task in simulation, without realising that, because patients vary, your practice in the initial stages will be supervised by someone more experienced. This will happen no matter how competent you feel. Expectations and self-appraisal are all implicated in the type of behaviours we exhibit, and how open to feedback we might or might not be. The skills and attributes needed for engaging with, and getting the most out of, clinical supervision include: communication skills, reflective ability, honesty and being open to feedback.

There are several models of clinical supervision, including: calling on an expert facilitator who has expertise in the problem area and can offer some solutions; one-to-one supervision where the individual meets with the supervisor alone; group supervision where a number of people meet with a supervisor; or using a supervisor from another discipline. Consideration of the model for supervision depends on whether the issue for discussion requires an expert, peer discussion could benefit all parties, a group holds similar concerns, an individual requires support or the issue is too sensitive to be aired in a group setting. Whichever is chosen, it is important to be clear about the aims of clinical supervision sessions.

Proctor (1986, cited in Hawkins and Shohet, 1989, p42) devised a framework that draws together the managerial, educative and support functions of clinical supervision. These are interpreted as follows:

1. Normative:
   a. Managerial function concerned with safe practice/developing standards;
   b. Ensures adherence to guidelines;
   c. Talking to more experienced practitioner who assists supervisee to work within these guidelines and meet standards.

151

2. Educational:

    a. Reflection and exploration;

    b. Enables supervisee to recognise strengths and weaknesses to develop;

    c. Relates theory to practice in a critical way.

3. Restorative:

    a. Supportive function of responding;

    b. Helps to understand how emotional involvement affects practice;

    c. Enables nurses to deal with their own reactions;

    d. Provides a workforce that can deal with critical incidents/problems.

Another framework offered by van Ooijen (2013) views getting the most out of clinical supervision as a developmental journey, as illustrated in Figure 8.1. The starting point is as a novice in the use and understanding of clinical supervision, but, as competence and knowledge increase, so practitioners start to become more independent in their thinking – which continues to grow with increasing expertise when engaging with clinical supervision.

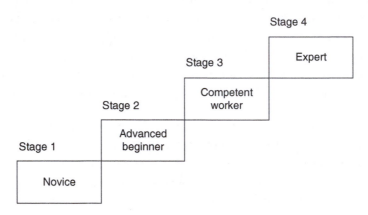

Figure 8.1 Developmental framework

(This diagram is taken from Els van Ooijen [2013] *Clinical Supervision Made Easy*, 2nd edn, and is reproduced with the kind permission of PCCS Books, Monmouth, p18.)

At the start of the journey, supervisees are highly motivated but lack insight and experience. As they progress to the next stage, they oscillate between being dependent on the supervisor and becoming more autonomous. At the stage after this, the supervisees have more confidence in their judgements, and at the end they act autonomously, with the supervision process becoming a two-way process in terms of reflective learning.

Clinical supervision, as noted at the start, offers the opportunity to develop reflective learning and deal with the emotional residues of caring work. According to Faugier and Butterworth (1994), clinical supervision is:

- sharing practice-based issues in confidence;
- getting feedback and guidance;
- developing professional knowledge through reflection;
- letting off steam;
- acknowledging feelings;
- feeling valued through supervisory support.

What clinical supervision is *not*:

- complaining;
- unstructured sharing of events;
- personal/family matters;
- being told what to do;
- disciplinary issues;
- other colleagues' performance.

Undertaking Activity 8.4 will help you apply these ideas in order to identify some suitable topics to bring to clinical supervision.

Activity 8.4   Critical thinking

Spend a little time thinking of topics that you think would be suitable to take to a clinical supervision session. Make a list so that you can reconsider how these might change during your working week. You can develop this further by choosing a trusted peer to offer peer supervision.

There is an outline answer to this activity at the end of the chapter.

It is important to reflect on a suitable topic well before a clinical supervision session in order to prioritise what is significant for your learning. According to Driscoll (2007), a clinical supervision session involves:

- *preparation*: reflecting on the topic you plan to bring;
- *settling in*: the clinical supervisor will help you to relax;
- *down to business*: you will be asked to present your issue concisely;
- *clarification and summarising*: the supervisor will clarify what is important;
- *closure*: the supervisor closes the session with action planning.

As you will have noticed, clinical supervision is focused on your learning through the topics that you bring. It is also time that is dedicated to you and therefore something that is very valuable and affirming. Making regular use of it as a healthcare practitioner can really help you to grow.

Chapter summary

This chapter has looked at several different reflective frameworks and ways of reflecting with others. The importance of others in stimulating the breadth of reflective knowledge has been emphasised because nursing interfaces with so many professions and this can enrich reflective processes. Through the scenarios and case studies you have been given an illustration of possible applications, with the activities offering you some guidance on identifying how you might proceed to incorporate some of these forms of reflection into your own practice and learning. How you start to record your reflections and write reflectively as another form of development is explored in the next chapter.

Activities and scenarios: Brief outline answers

Activity 8.1 Reflection on Sally's experience with death and dying (page 142)

Death, the accompanying rituals and how people feel about it have different cultural meanings. These may relate to belief systems and personal values. Belief systems may be religious or historically embedded in a culture. For the nurse, belief rituals and psychological aspects are the focus. In Scenario 8.1, cultural meaning for Sharon lies in her belief that people should not die alone. Historically, this has been a common value in nursing. Sally followed this direction because of the psychological, emotional bond she had developed with Amanda. Sally is more emotionally bound to the situation than Sharon. But Sharon is aware of the psychological residues for Sally and offers support, creating an encouraging culture for learning. It is hard to know what Amanda would have wanted, although there might have been some historical clues leading up to the event. For example, she might have preferred a relative or friend to be with her, and this might have been evident through her conversations about her life when she talked to Sally earlier on. However, if Sally's culture was markedly different to Amanda's it is likely that Sally might have struggled and needed further advice and knowledge. We need to consider what we mean by culture and how misleading assumptions can be. We often think of culture in terms of ethnicity, race, religion, etc., but we need to think of how varied our own culture is. It is imperative to understand the patient's wishes, but the contact suggested here is deeper than intellect. Turkel et al. (2018) and Watson (2008) suggest that caring is universal at a human level, that it transcends the barriers of culture. In Scenario 8.1 the impression is that, due to the contact Sally had developed with Amanda, they shared the same values and beliefs. Similarly, Sharon shared the perception that they had an understanding of what Amanda wanted at the end of her life and encouraged Sally to stay with her. Gerow et al. (2010, p124) found that nurses create a 'curtain of protection' to cope with their grieving, allowing them to support the dying patient. This appears to be what happened with Sally and Amanda. Gerow et al. (2010) also suggest that this 'curtain' bonds the nurse and patient in a special relationship, and that witnessing death is formative for the individual and will determine the type of curtain that is created. If you are at the start of the nursing programme, psychological aspects might be the most prominent, depending on your personal history and whether you have had dealings with death before. If you are experienced, you will have been exposed to the culture of nursing and will have developed coping mechanisms to help you deal with emotions. If you are very experienced, your history as a nurse will determine what you see as important, how you react and what kind of nursing culture you create. A risk would be if Sharon had negative experiences early in her career; she could respond differently to this situation and so could have been less satisfying for Sally's first exposure to death. Here, Sharon was sensitive to what she saw were Amanda's and Sally's needs to have a positive experience of death and dying. Pickersgill (2015, p64), in an interview with hospice nurses, summarises what many nurses think: *it is an enormous privilege to be with people at the end of life.* It is interesting to explore how elements of the NMC's Code (NMC, 2018b) come into play. Please read through the Code, paying particular attention to the section *Prioritise people* (items: 1.1–1.5, 2.1–2.6, 3.1–3.4, 4.1, 4.2, 4.4, 5.1, 5.3 and 5.5).

Activity 8.2 Reflections on Veronica's first day on a new placement (page 143)

The first issue in Scenario 8.2 is the initial impression that Greg's welcome makes. This first impression has stayed with her, making her feel valued and supported, counteracting the anxiety of the visit to Harry. The second issue is Veronica's shock at Harry's behaviour, which clearly is different to Veronica's values and beliefs. Greg could explore these further with her. Greg supports Veronica by sharing his thinking and decision-making with her. Veronica could enhance her understanding by sourcing information about the reasons for such behaviours. They could discuss how patient-centredness fits with a situation you find difficult to understand and how the NMC's Code (NMC, 2018b) can inform decisions. Please look up sections of the NMC's Code (NMC, 2018b) that apply to this scenario, for example, *Prioritise people* (items 1.1–1.3, 1.5, 2.1–2.5, 4.1, 4.3, 4.4, 5.1 and 5.4) and *Practise effectively* (items 7.1–7.4, 8.3, 8.4 and 10.1–10.6).

Activity 8.3 Reflection (pages 147–8)

You might identify placements such as radiology with offering collaboration with radiographers, rehabilitation areas with providing access to physiotherapists, occupational therapists and social workers, theatres with enabling connection with operating department practitioners, and women's health and day surgery arenas with offering an interface with midwifery. Equally, during your orientation weeks you will have access to other professionals such as those working with children, mental health and learning disabilities. All these offer opportunities for reflecting with others through multidisciplinary meetings, reflective learning groups and case conferences. Equally, at university you may be involved in joint learning with other health and social care students, and this could involve elements of reflection on professional identity and the contribution from different professions. Your action plan might identify how to become involved in some of these activities the next time you are on placement. You might have included thinking about with whom your practice has interfaced and what you have learned when talking in the classroom. Initial reflective questions might be the following:

- How does this profession's priorities interface with those of nurses?
- What, as a nurse practitioner, can I learn about this profession?
- How does knowledge of other professionals influence my practice now?

As an experienced practitioner you might have considered arranging opportunities for students to spend the day with professionals allied to your area. You might arrange for these professionals to undertake some teaching sessions in your area. A study by Esterhuizen and Kooijman (2001), exploring interprofessional schooling on moral decision-making, found that communication improved between disciplines and that issues were discussed earlier. The nursing role to initiate discussion with the multidisciplinary team should not be underestimated as we have always assumed the role of patient advocate.

Activity 8.4 Critical thinking (page 153)

The kind of topics that you might have thought about could include:

- professional issues;
- exploring learning and development options;
- work-related interpersonal relationships;
- ethical/legal issues;
- work experiences, both positive and negative;
- skills development;
- managerial development.

You may have identified some new ideas when reflecting with your trusted peers and might have been open to their suggestions because you trusted them. However, although such guided reflection is useful for opening up your critical thinking, you will need an experienced guide to reach any depth.

Further reading

Freshwater, D, Walsh, E and Esterhuizen, P (2007) Models of effective and reflective teaching and learning for best practice. In Bishop, V (ed.), *Clinical Supervision in Practice: Some questions, answers and guidelines for professionals in health and social care*, 2nd edn. Basingstoke: Palgrave Macmillan.

This book will help you to understand the importance of clinical supervision to the individual, to the patient/client and to the organisation of healthcare, and provide you with practical knowledge around implementation.

Higgs, J, Richardson, B and Abrandt Dahlgren, M (eds) (2004) *Developing Practice Knowledge for Health Professionals*. Edinburgh: Butterworth Heinemann.

This book will help you to understand how craft knowledge develops and how this relates to different forms of knowledge.

Johns, C (2010) *Guided Reflection: A narrative approach to advancing professional practice*, 2nd edn. Chichester: Wiley-Blackwell.

This book explains guided reflection through a number of exemplars and the author's practice.

Milne, D (2009) *Evidence-Based Clinical Supervision: Principles and practice*. Oxford: British Psychological Society and Blackwell.

This book presents the evidence base for using clinical supervision techniques and is especially useful for experienced practitioners in developing their practice.

van Ooijen, E (2013) *Clinical Supervision Made Easy*, 2nd edn. Monmouth: PCCS Books.

This book explains clinical supervision in a way that is easy to understand.

Useful websites

www.supervisionandcoaching.com

This website offers resources for explaining different forms of reflection and for undertaking clinical supervision.

Chapter 9 Reflective writing

Chapter aims

After reading this chapter you will be able to:

- define writing reflectively;
- understand the principles of confidentiality and reflective writing;
- undertake personal reflective writing, such as keeping a reflective journal;
- undertake personal development planning;
- write reflectively in assignments as appropriate;
- record guided reflection.

Introduction

Scenario 9.1: Talula's creative reflection

Talula was in the second year of her nursing programme and undertaking a module which involved reflecting on the quality of person-centred care and compassion. Talula was required to use creative methods to produce an assignment about the strategies she had used to enhance person-centred care and what she had learned about herself through the process. As Talula was a naturally creative person she was excited about this assignment and began to think about how she might approach it. She considered writing a short story about a recent patient encounter on placement, but when she read it through it was too long. Instead Talula decided to write a poem that captured what she thought were the key aspects of person-centred care in the case. Talula was pleased with her poem and sent the draft to her tutor for comment and feedback.

Talula's tutor was impressed with the poem and gave Talula positive feedback. However, she also indicated that the element of what Talula had learned about herself as a nurse working in person-centred ways was missing. Talula thought about this and considered how she might weave this element into her poem. Talula realised that she had not really made use of any narrative structure and decided to read more about this. She concluded that connecting reading with thinking and doing were important components. After reading about narrative structure Talula went for a walk to help make sense of things and found that she needed a few days to think through what she needed, but also wanted, to do. A few days later she began her poem again, this time including a refrain that enabled her to weave in her own thoughts more explicitly. It was quite challenging because Talula was aware that the whole poem was about her thoughts, how she viewed the patient and the way she interpreted patient-centredness. However, when Talula received the results of her assignment, she was delighted to receive a high mark and extremely positive feedback.

The example above shows that even playful forms of writing reflectively require depth of thinking with regard to content and how to represent your ideas coherently and effectively. Besides being a vehicle that allows you to consider your experiences in a different way, learning to write reflectively will equip you with the relevant ethical and analytical ability to benefit from your practice experiences. To do this you will need to look back on significant incidents, examine surrounding concepts and engage in an analysis of them.

This chapter explores the purpose of reflective writing in relation to the standards of proficiency required by nursing regulators. You will be introduced to a variety of techniques and encouraged to try out some different exercises to help to develop this skill. In particular, you will be invited to begin personal development planning related to your reflective log. How to write reflectively in assignments is also developed in more detail.

Writing reflectively

Writing about your experiences will help you to make sense of them so that your understanding lasts and contributes to your life-long learning. Reflection about experiences may be articulated in different ways when you are speaking or writing about them. Speaking about situations tends to be exploratory as your thoughts are put into words. However, writing about the circumstances is very powerful as you place your thoughts outside of yourself. Reading and re-reading your writing allow you to 'objectify' your own thoughts and behaviour, and it is fascinating to experience how differently we can view a situation, depending on our state of mind at the time. We tend to focus on negative or unpleasant things when reflecting, and reflective writing and re-reading these accounts allow us to view the situation from a less emotionally engaged position, in retrospect. Putting things in black and white may sometimes be subject to concerns with the presentation and the scrutiny of an invisible audience. It is important, when starting out to write reflectively, that concerns about who might read it are reduced, in order for you to be able to be honest and authentic in *your* reflective evaluation and writing about *your* experience. Bolton (2014) suggests that, like Alice in Wonderland, it is important to be open to uncertainty and new experience in playful ways. In other words, *to venture outside the firmly boundaried inner self into a place of exploration* (Bolton, 2014, p11). Writing in this way demands breadth and depth, and a commitment to explore and not be afraid of what you might find out. Starting such a writing journey means writing in formative and unfinished ways, first capturing your deepest thoughts and feelings as they start to surface. Consider the following examples of reflective writing from the student nurse (Joe) and ward manager (Ross) perspective, then answer the questions in Activity 9.1.

Scenario 9.2: Joe and Ross's confrontation

Student reflection example (Joe)

I am a student nurse on a mental health nursing preparation programme and am having difficulties with my practice supervisor Ross. I have had some personal issues resulting in my being unwell and, therefore, needing time off sick. I phoned the ward and left a message for Ross. However, when I came back to work Ross told me (in front of other staff) that it was unprofessional not to notify the ward that I wasn't coming in, and this seemed to be becoming a habit. He said he would have to report this to the university.

I feel persecuted, bullied and upset because, despite telling Ross I had informed the ward, he is still threatening to tell the university. This is compromising my learning because I am now anxious around Ross. I spoke to the link tutor, Elaine, who arranged a meeting with Ross and me. The meeting with Elaine and Ross helped me to explain that I had contacted the ward and left a message and also helped clarify our expectations of each other. I was able to say how anxious this episode had left me feeling and to plan a way forward with Ross.

I came away from the meeting feeling more positive because Elaine had highlighted that on busy wards messages are not always passed on; therefore, I feel she believed me. But I am unsure whether Ross will adhere to the actions of a communication pathway that we discussed. I am still a bit on edge around him and focused on not getting things wrong. As a consequence, I am reluctant to try new things and expand my scope of practice. My relationship with Ross is one of wary collaboration, which does not feel like a good learning relationship. He does not appear to notice. Surely a practice supervisor should be able to perceive the quality of a learning relationship?

If I were in Ross's shoes I would welcome my student back by asking them how they were first and then finding out what had happened, in a confidential space. This would allow issues to emerge in a supportive atmosphere and enable us both to manage emotions. What this has taught me is the type of support I would like to espouse, namely, supportive, nurturing, empowering, and I have therefore kept this reflection to return to. I plan to discuss this further with Ross at our next meeting.

Practitioner reflection example (Ross)

I am supporting a student nurse called Joe. I have only been a practice supervisor for six months. The ward is busy, and we are currently short staffed. I am also supporting two other students. I was cross that Joe had not turned up on shift yesterday and had not notified me. Does he realise the implications for the patient and staff if he does not come on duty? When Joe arrived back on duty today I asked him crossly why he had not notified me that he would be absent and whether he realised how unprofessional such behaviour was. I could see by the look on his face that Joe was angry, but I was too busy to follow this up. Since then I have had a meeting with Joe and a tutor from the university called Elaine. Joe explained that he had rung the ward and left a message with Tom – a new member of staff. I remember the ward was busy yesterday and the message must have got lost. We discussed ways this might be avoided in future by using a communication book on the ward.

(Continued)

(Continued)

I feel guilty now for having a go at Joe without establishing the facts first. I realise I am a person who needs to get on with things before I forget them, and that I can be impatient at times. I do expect Joe to be more assertive in his needs as a student. I think at our next meeting it might be useful to start by discussing how things are going for Joe, and ways in which I can support him further and gain some feedback on my style of supporting learners. I recognise that I still have a lot to learn about this and it might be helpful for me to work with the practice assessor to gain more knowledge.

Activity 9.1   Reflection

After reading the two examples of early reflective writing above, answer the following questions:

- What is Joe's focus for reflection?
- What is Ross's focus for reflection?
- Are any further actions planned?
- If you were either Joe or Ross, how could you add depth to the reflection?

There are outline answers to these questions at the end of the chapter.

Reasons for reflective writing may vary, but the result is that you can begin to feel more empowered as you take control of your own development and learning, and you can come to a more positive view of difficult situations. However, the actual process can be emotionally demanding in what it reveals about you as a person and perhaps about others too. There are many reasons for undertaking reflective writing. These include:

- to log and record personal and professional experience and development;
- to help make sense of emotionally charged situations;
- to record other forms of reflection, such as guided reflection;
- to identify and plan career progression;
- to provide evidence of learning;
- to fulfil assignment requirements;
- to deepen understanding;
- for your own interest.

Read Scenario 9.3 to consider what opportunity it presents for reflective writing.

Scenario 9.3: Faheed's experience of group cultural differences

Faheed was in the first year of his mental health nursing programme. His peer group at university comprised a diverse range of students from a variety of backgrounds and different professional pathways. They were studying a collaborative module that required them to develop patches of writing reflecting on professional values that they worked on in groups and to present their writing to the class for peer feedback at the development stage.

Faheed recognised that there were problems with group dynamics when they were at a break and some people complained about the task and having to learn with other pathway students. Faheed spoke up, saying how important it was for professions to understand each other and work together for the good of the patient. He related a personal example of a family member recovering from serious injury with the help of different professions working together. The group began to see the relevance of the learning activity and returned to the class and task with more enthusiasm.

Activity 9.2   Reflection

- What learning might Faheed take from this situation?
- How might Faheed compose his patch text about different professions working together?

There is an outline answer to these questions at the end of the chapter.

Ehrmann (2005) identifies that disruptive and aggressive behaviours arise from power struggles and a sense of competitiveness. This behaviour may result in a failure to control 'self' in practice, which has implications for patients and staff. Team relationships in any situation are always influenced by the personalities, psychological states and cultures of the people involved. Xu and Davidhizar (2005) suggest that there are cultural differences in communication patterns that can lead to misinterpretations and breakdowns. Western and European culture follows an individualistic pattern, whereas Eastern and African cultures favour group patterns. Students sometimes feel disempowered, and reluctant to share their needs for fear of discrimination (Dalton, 2005). When faced by a dominant group in the classroom, it might appear to be difficult to have your voice heard. If others' responses are not encouraging it is easy to become discouraged and silenced.

Numerous authors. including Hutchinson et al. (2006), Farrell (2001) and Freshwater (2000), have discussed the phenomenon of workplace bullying and horizontal violence. Although it is not the intention here to focus on the potentially less positive experiences of study and work, the scenarios of Joe and Ross, and Faheed, do have the ring of bullying and victimisation. It is, therefore, prudent to pause at this point to consider the implications of this behaviour within a work or university environment because this may well form part of your reflections and reflective writing as you progress through your career.

Activity 9.3   Reflection

Please read the articles by Hutchinson et al. (2006), Farrell (2001) and Freshwater (2000) and then consider the ideas you had concerning Activities 9.1 and 9.2. Perhaps you could jot down a few thoughts on the following points:

- How do you view Scenarios 9.2 and 9.3 after reading these articles?
- Has your view and interpretation of the scenario changed through reading the three papers? If so, please jot down how your perception has changed, and whether you would offer different insights and advice when asked to comment.
- Do any of the issues raised in the articles resonate with your experiences in either the university or the practice setting? If so, how did you address the issues when they arose, and could you address the situation differently after reading these articles?

This activity is based on your reading the suggested articles. The full references can be found at the end of the chapter. However, as this is your own reflection, there is no outline answer.

Whichever setting we work in, it will always be necessary for people from different cultures to learn to adapt to each other in order to communicate effectively for patient care. We should be mindful that, when talking about cultures, we do not always refer to ethnicity, language, religion, etc., but should also be aware that gender, gender identity, age, sexual orientation, geographical location, etc. are all elements of culture that could result in different ideas and behaviour in particular situations. Part of the learning process is to bridge these divides and develop opportunities. Curiosity and reflection about difference, commonality and inclusion are core concepts in interpersonal communication, respect and acceptance – accepting and respecting 'the other' means first to accept and respect 'self'. Development in this area can be achieved by continued reflection on what is happening and potential reasons why, and by considering alternatives. Writing reflectively will help you to deal with these types of situations and with the implementation of ideas, and is a powerful way of gaining *empowerment* within such situations. However, as our experiences inevitably involve others too, it is important to recognise, within reflective writing, personal responsibility and accountability to maintain the anonymity and confidentiality of others. We will consider this in more detail in the next section.

The principles of confidentiality in reflective writing

Confidentiality is a key ethical issue in professional practice in terms of what is written and discussed (Nursing and Midwifery Council [NMC], 2018a). Patient confidentiality is prioritised, but corporate confidentiality is not always as easily considered. The Caldicott Committee recommended that all items of information relating to an individual should be treated as potentially capable of identifying them, and be appropriately protected to safeguard confidentiality (Department of Health [DH], 1997). Confidentiality means keeping information private. Corporate confidentiality means that institutions and organisations are also entitled to have their business kept private. This may be achieved by using a pseudonym and removal of any identifiers of the issues being written about. It is important when using someone else's information (such as a patient's case) to gain their consent for its use.

There are concerns about the morality of using interpreted information about someone as a learning resource (Dawber, 2012; Hargreaves, 1997; McCarthy et al., 2016). This applies to information about clients, or others, when writing reflectively, and creates a professional conduct issue and an ethical dilemma. One method is to attempt to 'bracket' identifiers, thus focusing on the core issues. By stripping away all descriptors that cause distraction, the foundation issues can emerge and be decided on. Johns' (2013) framework, as discussed in Chapter 4, offers an alternative by examining background philosophy, theory and problem presentation, as well as interpretation of reality, role and self-awareness in the form of questions, eliminating the necessity for descriptors. Background philosophy relates to what kind of values and beliefs may be present in assumptions made about the problem, whereas theory is about the kind of framework that surrounds thinking about the problem. These will both be involved in how a problem is presented and in the interpretation of the reality of the problem. Questioning your own role reflectively and developing self-awareness in relation to the problem is necessary, and this might be a useful model to try.

Activity 9.4   Reflection

Using Johns' (2013) questions of philosophy, theory, problem presentation, interpretation of reality, role and self-awareness, write a reflective account of the episode relating to your practice that you identified in Activity 9.3.

As this activity relates to your practice, there is no outline answer at the end of the chapter.

Please be mindful that using student and client knowledge needs to be ethically considerate and sensitive, focusing on issues in an evaluative and analytical manner, and examining personal parameters of responsibility. This applies not only to reflections on clinical experiences, but also classroom discussions, group work or any other joint activity. This is something that you need to consider when you write reflectively, regardless of whether or not you intend your writing to be seen by others. It is advisable not to focus on others in your reflections because they are not present to argue their case, or discuss issues with you in person; it is better to focus on issues, rather than people, and how an issue affected you and how you addressed it. This means that others' confidentiality is assured and that your and their professional roles are ethically protected (Brockbank and McGill, 2007).

Read Scenario 9.4 and answer the questions in Activity 9.5, to help you think of how you might approach these issues.

Scenario 9.4: Mia's reflection on collaborative learning

Mia is a registered nurse who had trained overseas. She was working in a renal unit where two third-year nurses, Josh and Ray, were currently completing their placements. Mia had recently begun an academic development course, which taught her how to search for information and complete academic assignments, in order to prepare her for going on to study a programme that would allow her to supervise and assess students in practice. Mia was anxious because she was having difficulty grasping the principles of reflection (something she was not used to because she had completed an exam-based course for her basic nursing education). Mia had completed a formative piece of work reflecting on what she had learned on the programme so far, but the feedback from her tutor had indicated that she had failed substantially because she had not maintained confidentiality or reflected adequately. Mia was confused. She had identified the type of unit she worked in, as well as the *trust* and where she was studying, but she had not named any of the patients. She had described her learning and what she wanted to do. Mia decided to ask Josh to help her, because he seemed to know a lot about reflection whenever she spoke about it at work. She was worried about 'losing face' with her tutor.

Mia asked Josh if he could explain how he reflected so that she could see what she was not doing. Josh asked Mia to think about her arrival in the trust from the perspective of how she felt at the time and how she felt about it now. As Mia was describing this event from the different time perspectives, Josh asked her various questions, which he wrote down with her answers. At the end he asked Mia to read back what he had recorded from their dialogue. Mia was amazed at how Josh had captured her experience in a few words, but also how the questions had made her think differently about things. She decided to write about this process that evening and asked if Josh would look at it for her the next day.

Mia rewrote the piece of dialogue by including how she felt her knowledge had changed and how building relationships with people had made things easier. She was careful not to include Josh's name, but to relate the issue of developing knowledge through working and learning collaboratively with students. Mia did make some critical points about how her arrival could have been facilitated better.

Mia showed the piece she had written to Josh the next day. Josh made some helpful comments and identified a book that Mia might find helpful to inform her thinking about reflection. Mia felt more affirmed.

Activity 9.5   Reflection

- In Scenario 9.4, how did Mia breach confidentiality within her formative piece of writing?
- What might be the consequences for her and what might be the consequences for Josh if he breached confidentiality in a similar way in his written work?

There are outline answers to these questions at the end of the chapter.

Collaborative learning between those who are already qualified and students is a valuable process. This is especially useful when considering issues of confidentiality, to help the student understand the parameters of accountability and why qualified staff and practice supervisors might see situations differently or become anxious. Stripping away all descriptors could contribute to losing the context, so realistic description within consent might be a more reliable, as well as ethical, option. We now move on to consider the role of personal reflective writing as a part of this process.

Personal reflective writing

Reflection in nursing has a dual function in supporting learning, but also supporting the individual. It requires considerable confidence and courage to acknowledge limitations and deficits, and a degree of insight to admit these to ourselves. According to Bolton (2014, p116), 'through the mirror' writing can facilitate:

- gaining perspective;
- giving confidential and relatively safe access;
- releasing power to take more responsibility for actions;
- using narrative [offers] accurate observation, metaphor and critique.

From this perspective, such writing is always temporal and evolving, and may generate unexpected ideas. For example, when thinking about what caring means to you, you might suddenly remember when you were ill in bed at home as a child, and how wretched and unwell you felt. You might vividly *feel* the rumpled sheets and the resulting discomfort, the clamminess of the temperature, and how lonely you felt because all your friends were at school. This might make you revise more glib ideas of caring into something much more personal.

Making use of art forms such as poetry, as used by Talula in Scenario 9.1, or scenes of a play, may greatly increase the fluidity of expression and help deal with emotions that are sometimes difficult by creating *cathartic* expression through the writing. Some people find it helpful to create a collage of pictures, cut out from magazines, that symbolise their ideas and/or feelings and then, once visually portrayed, to write about the issue on which they need to focus. Other people use dance and movement to express their ideas and emotions and, in doing this, make their abstract thoughts more tangible before writing them down (McCarthy et al., 2016). Writing in this way develops a different articulation which can be empowering because you, and the reader, are trying to make sense of your personal experience, to gain control of the emotions and the issues involved in the reflection.

Richardson (1997) and, more recently, Coleman and Willis (2015) invite the reflective writer to find new forms of expression. To empower ourselves requires coming to know ourselves as being more than a professional identity (think of the personal biography that we spoke about in Chapter 3). It is in knowing ourselves that we can hope to come to know our 'becoming' as well (Chan and Schwind, 2006). Poetic expression can express a unique part of who you are, and does not necessarily have to follow any particular rules. Rather, it provides an opportunity for the playfulness described earlier in this chapter by Bolton (2014) as an essential part of going through the mirror, rather than becoming fixated with its surface. Poetry may not be something with which you feel comfortable, and it is not essential to use this form of expression, but try it out and you may surprise yourself. Remember, no one needs to see your writing. An example of poetry follows.

> *What do you see when you look at me?*
>
> *A caring nurse or a man alone;*
>
> *What do you see when you look at me?*
>
> *A capable helper or someone losing his home;*
>
> *What do you see when you look at me?*
>
> *Someone missing class or trying to phone;*
>
> *What do you see when you look at me?*
>
> *See the person, see the problem, see ME.*

This could have been how Joe might have started writing about his frustration in the student reflection earlier. Undertaking the next activity will offer you the opportunity to express yourself differently.

Activity 9.6   Reflection

Think of something relating to your personal development that is very significant to you. Spend a little time reflecting on the situation or issue. Now try to write a reflection about it in the form of a poem or as scenes of a play. Re-read this and consider what response and insights this form of expression elicits.

As this activity is based on your personal experiences, there is an outline answer to only part of this activity at the end of the chapter.

Personal writing may never be seen by another person, because it is a form of a diary that records your deepest impressions and considerations about what you are thinking and doing. This differs marginally from a reflective journal, which we consider next.

The reflective journal

Although personal reflective writing can be cathartic and *catalytic*, helping you let go of your emotions and achieve deep exploration (Driscoll, 2007), there also needs to be reflection on how your role might develop as healthcare progresses and you develop professionally in the course of your career. Logging reflective entries within a reflective journal helps keep track of what you are learning and your practice experiences, including those you encounter through your preparation programme. In addition, consistent writing helps you to consider assessment, feedback and practice in terms of your whole experience and can, therefore, be a powerful way to integrate theory and practice. This approach, often introduced as part of the nursing programme, is imperative to professional life-long learning and will be used in maintaining a professional portfolio and revalidation as a registered nurse (NMC, 2017).

Example of a reflective log entry

Self-assessing experience

I had taken on teaching a course that was new to me, and the first session had gone well. However, by the third session the group were clearly confused by the advice I was giving them. I had checked with the module leader regarding the assignment, but I found their explanation was as woolly as the written guidelines. A number of students e-mailed the module leader directly and I was copied into the replies, which gave some clarity. At the next session I was able to give some concrete examples of what they might want to write about. However, overall my teaching of this aspect of the module was badly evaluated, which was disappointing.

Main points identified from reflection on the experience

- I had not been proactive, when agreeing to teach on the module, to ensure that I understood what the learning outcomes for the module were and how the assessment related to the outcomes.
- I did not communicate my understanding clearly to the module leader when I asked for advice on the guidelines. I should have asked for further clarification.
- I had not told the students at the start that this was the first time I was teaching the module. I should have done this because, in hindsight, we could have worked better together to clarify the guidelines with the module leader. Using the knowledge of other, experienced tutors of the module would also have been helpful.

Learning points

- I need to be prepared to ask for help from both colleagues and students, to work together.
- I need to be open to identifying alternative strategies, which could aid learning.
- I need to acknowledge to myself and the other person that I do not understand the information being given.

How will this learning be applied in the future?

- I will ensure that I have a good understanding of what the module entails and how the assessment relates to the learning outcomes.
- I will address my feelings associated with asking for help and further explanation.
- I will tell students if I am new to teaching a module and work with them in less formal ways.

As indicated earlier, a registered nurse is also expected to keep a portfolio of evidence to demonstrate learning for the regulatory body. At its simplest level, maintaining a reflective journal is a good starting point for demonstrating what and how you are learning. How you interact with different people is also important, because nursing is about communicating with a variety of different people. Group dynamics are often key to learning and need to be given early attention (Jacques, 2000). Reflection and self-development play an increasing part in this process. By undertaking Activity 9.7, you will help yourself get started with logging such experiences.

Activity 9.7   Reflection

Think of a recent experience (this could be from within the university or from practice). Now write about the following using one of the models discussed in Chapter 4:

- Describe the experience.
- What essential factors contributed to this experience and are there significant features?

When you have kept your journal for a week or so, revisit it and consider the following:

- What are the themes emerging from the journal entries?
- What sense do you make of this and using what evidence?

As this activity is based on your personal experiences, there is an outline answer to only part of this activity at the end of the chapter.

It is human to want to place 'blame' with someone else if things do not go according to plan, or if we feel embarrassed by our mistake or oversight. Expressing dissatisfaction with others is known as a form of 'othering' that can remove responsibility and personal accountability to address the situation. It is very important as a professional to identify and acknowledge when this happens. If you find yourself starting to use 'othering', there is also the possibility, through reflection, to consciously reject this path (Freshwater, 2000). Reflection and open dialogue are the best options to support trust in fragile circumstances, but could also be confronting for the less confident. Writing in your reflective journal how you intend to deal with the situation is a good starting point for taking proactive action, rather than leaving things to drift and relationships to suffer. The reflective journal is a useful tool for evaluating your strengths, weaknesses, interests and areas for development through reviewing such difficult issues and the emerging themes, as discussed at the start of this section. This review can inform your personal development planning, and is discussed next.

Personal development planning

As early as 1997, Scanlan and Chernomas discussed how reflection creates vulnerability in terms of exposing thinking and practice to criticism, and self-concept to realignment. This has been supported, more recently, by the work of Padykula (2017) and Ruyak et al. (2017), who suggest that reflection and self-awareness takes courage, commitment, cognitive insight and emotional resilience. Planning involves reflecting on strengths and areas for improvement, and the interplay between the past and the future, to inform, shape implementation strategies and translate these into concrete actions. We perhaps need to refocus at this point by reminding ourselves that reflection here is a learning strategy, leading to personal and/or professional development. As such the action that results from such processes, again, requires courage and commitment to try something new and to acknowledge the possibility of being wrong, but still to recognise the learning gain. This means making use of past learning experiences to interpret present practice and knowledge when writing reflectively, and for personal development planning, projecting outcomes and perhaps further learning into the future. This is an important point to consider when thinking about your learning contracts and whether they are product, rather than process, focused.

A product-focused plan may be promoted by time constraints, but then arguably does not achieve the purpose, raising questions of accountability for both practice supervisors and learners. Feedback is an important component of reviewing progress, in that it provides evaluative information that can be reflected on and incorporated into planning future action and learning. It is important to have thought through what you are attempting to achieve, and your potential commitment, in order to ensure that you can deliver consistently and equitably on the activities. Table 9.1 gives some headings that you might like to consider as part of your personal development planning.

What are my learning and development needs?	What do I want to gain from this development?	What support do I need and from whom?	Evaluation/review
Student: I need to learn more about drug administration Learning objective: By week 10 of my placement, I am able to explain and administer six (6) medications in terms of: • Action • Effect/indication • Route • Dose • Common side effects (In relation to a patient) • Risks (In relation to a patient) • Drug calculation (In relation to a patient) • Correct management, administration and storage of the medication • Safe administration (in relation to an identified individual patient with specification of the route used)	1. To be more proficient and have greater knowledge of different drug groups 2. To be aware of, and recognise, risks and side effects of the medications I administer	1. My practice supervisor to give me opportunity to practice 2. Access to formulary books 3. Create opportunities to discuss the medications I see in practice, with my practice supervisor, in relation to actual patients	1. Review progress with my practice supervisor at the second and third meeting dates 2. Evaluate with my practice supervisor whether I have achieved the learning objectives set at the start of the placement 3. Set learning objectives for my next placement that allow me to develop my skills and knowledge

What are my learning and development needs?	What do I want to gain from this development?	What support do I need and from whom?	Evaluation/review
Practitioner: I need to learn more about how to build positive learning relationships	1. Be able to support a range of students by creating a positive learning environment	1. Organise an experienced practice supervisor who will support and advise me in developing a positive learning environment	1. Evaluate whether the student is settled in the clinical environment and whether they feel comfortable and safe on the placement

(Continued)

Table 9.1 (Continued)

What are my learning and development needs?	What do I want to gain from this development?	What support do I need and from whom?	Evaluation/review
Learning objective: By week 10 of supporting a student on placement, I am able to: • Demonstrate understanding factors influencing how students integrate into, and learn from, practice settings • Provide constructive support to allow student transition from one learning environment to another • Have working relationships to support learning for the entry to register	2. Develop awareness of and understand which factors influence my student's learning 3. Develop a plan of action to help the student adapt to a new placement 4. Be confident that I have supported the student to develop professional and interprofessional relationships	2. Organise an experienced practice supervisor such as a practice assessor to support and advise me in the assessment process 3. Discuss which skills the student has achieved in previous placements and what they need to achieve in this placement 4. Discuss how the student learns and what they expect from my practice supervision	2. Review the student's progress every three weeks and establish whether they have sufficient opportunity to achieve their learning objectives 3. Ask the student for specific feedback on my practice supervisor style 4. Final student placement evaluation

Table 9.1 Headings to organise your personal development

It is important that you identify learning objectives that you want to achieve from a situation and ensure that you understand what is expected of you. It is equally important that you articulate your expectations when going into practice, or when being asked to complete independent study. This is helpful for you because it means that (a) you have clarity in terms of expectations, (b) it is beneficial for your practice or academic supervisor because they are clear as to your level of understanding, and (c) most importantly, you are taking control of your learning by being proactive. Undertaking Activity 9.8 offers you an opportunity to think reflectively about these issues.

Activity 9.8   Critical thinking

Think about your next placement, or next year, if appropriate. If you are an experienced practitioner, think about your next appraisal. Now consider the following questions:

- What are your strengths?
- What are your weaknesses?
- How do you know this (are there any aspects that make you feel uncertain)?
- What are you planning to do about this?
- What, from reflection, do you need to take forward (what opportunities will this offer)?

Now write a reflective account to draw these (SWOT) elements into a whole as evidence for your portfolio.

As this activity is based on your personal experiences, there is an outline answer to only part of this activity at the end of the chapter.

Personal development planning is an important way to develop agency in your own learning and ensure that it is linked to your needs. This principle continues throughout your career and often a personal learning plan forms the basis of annual appraisal meetings. As a registered healthcare professional, it is incorporated into professional validation and triennial reviews.

In order to provide evidence of your personal development, you also need to write about it within formal assignments, whether you are a student on a preparation programme or an experienced practitioner undertaking study at university. We now consider reflective writing in assignments.

Reflective writing in assignments

When discussing reflective writing it is worth considering an interesting point made by Hargreaves (2004, p200) in which she suggests that we generally produce three types of reflective narrative:

- *Valedictory*, where we save a 'bad situation' and come out victorious at the end;
- *Condemnatory*, where a situation goes wrong and we cannot resolve it, but emerge feeling dissatisfied and, possibly, guilty;
- *Redemptive* narrative, where we respond inappropriately to a situation, but then redeem ourselves, suggesting that we have improved our practice.

These three narrative types may develop unconsciously, and it is worth trying to recognise whether you favour a particular approach as we move into discussing reflective writing in assignments.

Nursing's professional voice is situated in practice and practitioners 'know nursing' as an insider. By understanding the process and cyclical nature of healthcare, the contextual decision-making and educational practice make this 'inside knowledge' easier to articulate. In contrast, an academic voice in nursing can feel less straightforward, requiring intellectual effort to negotiate different viewpoints, parameters and theoretical models. Reflection, as we have already discussed, is a valuable part of the learning and teaching process, but it needs to be purposeful and carefully integrated within curricula to achieve relevant and credible learning. Threatening or contentious experiences may be ignored or translated into more acceptable versions to meet course requirements or role expectations, rather than make sense of processes. For example, it may be difficult to write about mistakes or less positive placement experiences for fear of punitive measures or penalties. There is an ethical tension if issues appear in reflective accounts from practice that appears unsound, or unsafe, because academic staff are also professionally bound to escalate concerns while balancing confidentiality with the duty of care to the student. There must be a documented process to follow that is clear to all parties, with well-defined outcomes for the process. Within this, academic and practice responsibility can be shared more readily to enable learning and build your self-confidence. Naturally, this can happen only in an open and trusting environment that calls for clear intercollegiate communication and sound professional values from all parties concerned.

Marking and, therefore, producing reflective writing in assignments are focused on the breadth and depth of the reflective content. This follows a continuum of whether written reflection and the conclusions reached are perceptive and significant with convincing conclusions, or whether they are superficial and lack relevance. Advancing to the further reaches of this continuum requires moving beyond the description of reflection and offering perceptive reflection, which ranges beyond the immediate context to include subtle thought and originality. This involves:

- considering what theoretical concepts are active in the situation;
- any unique features that the situation is demonstrating;
- what your view is, based on experience and reflection – give examples;
- keeping the focus on *your* practice and not generalising to some abstract generic view.

A brief example of a reflective paragraph that might be part of reflective writing in assignments is offered below.

Example of reflective writing in assignments

Completing the long-term conditions module has made me think again about how I approach and think about people with long-term and often complex illnesses. I realise that I am often focused on the task within the context of providing that specific care, and forget about the patient's experience and their expertise. It can become easy to get caught up in problem solving and leave them out. I find that I don't include the patient in the decision-making because I don't want to give them the impression that I'm uncertain or lack knowledge and skill in that particular area. I'm also aware that thinking only theoretically and cognitively separates me from important subjective and intuitive elements. I'm afraid that, in this way, the care that I provide can become objectified rather than me responding to the person. I know that I need to communicate my decision-making to the patient so that they are included, can offer their insights and expert experience from living with their condition and, consequently, be part of the solution. I will revisit person-centred care, shared decision-making and partnership literature, and make a conscious effort to include patients in my assessment and decision-making. I will discuss my plan of action with my practice supervisor, ask that they observe me with patients and provide me with specific feedback.

It sometimes helps to analyse reflection more deeply through guided reflection, as discussed in Chapter 8. When you are involved in guided reflection it is important to record the learning that this generates, in order to ensure that it is captured and not lost. We now consider how this is another form of reflective writing.

Recording guided reflection

Guided reflection can help address some of the ethical issues identified earlier around student vulnerability. This is achieved by using a partnership approach between student and practice/academic supervisor, to set clear outcomes for the issue and provide support during the process. The issue of a reconstructed past remains challenging, although careful questioning of and attentive listening to yourself, as well as questioning and active listening by the reflective guide, may facilitate this. In order to record guided reflection, the following pro forma is offered as a template, based on the one provided in Chapter 1.

PRO FORMA FOR DOCUMENTING GUIDED REFLECTION

Practice-based experience:

Main points identified from reflection on the experience:

Main points identified from guided exploration of the experience:

Learning points:

How will this learning be applied in practice?

Professional development achieved?

Chapter summary

Often reflection also dissolves in the reality of everyday work and life. Holism is achieved by embedding a continuous cycle of experimentation and review through reflective writing. Reflection is an art that requires insight and self-awareness, and it will take longer than the time allocated for a programme to develop fully because it is an aspect of professional life-long learning. Writing is one way to start embedding the process. The activities in this chapter have provided different opportunities to expand your writing and develop different techniques that could generate further reflective insights.

Activities and scenarios: Brief outline answers

Activity 9.1 Reflection on Joe and Ross's confrontation (page 162)

Joe focuses on his feelings and the impact on his learning. He has thought of what Ross could do differently and how he might respond if he were a practice supervisor.

Ross considers his and Joe's feelings and the causes. He has considered how his actions contributed to the current situation and what he can do about it.

Joe and Ross have planned further action, but neither has considered what the consequences might be. Further analysis could add depth to the reflection and include considering how the actions and influence of others and events could influence future behaviour.

Things that you may have thought about in terms of how Joe and Ross could develop their reflection further could have been:

- Joe could explore why he feels persecuted and victimised by the situation. Where does this come from (his biography)? What risks are involved in maintaining this behaviour? Could this (rather than Ross) be limiting his development on the ward? Which learning objectives could Joe formulate to overcome this feeling? How could Joe apply feedback guidelines to the situation? What could be his aims of a meeting with Ross?
- Ross could reflect on several issues. He could reflect on his strategies for coping with stress and how he sets his boundaries: why he accepted responsibility for three students and team leadership when he has little experience? Another area could be his impatience and his perfectionism. A third area might be his communication strategy as practice supervisor and role-model – issues about emotional intelligence and power could inform his reflection in this area.

Activity 9.2 Reflection on Faheed's experience of group cultural differences (page 163)

- Faheed might sense tensions within the group and who the leaders of the group are. He might recognise with whom he should discuss the group dynamic to achieve the best outcome. This might suggest to Faheed that he has leadership potential.
- Faheed might have learned about his communication and assertiveness skills by how his interaction had inspired the group. This could have increased his confidence.
- He might have identified how to minimise barriers between different professions. Faheed's patch text might have said something like:

'My uncle was injured in an accident. He was ventilated for 4 days in intensive care and then transferred to a ward. He was discharged 3 weeks later but needed help at home for another 2 weeks. The professionals involved in his recovery included doctors, nurses, physiotherapists, occupational therapists and community nurses. I saw the different professions working closely together in the intensive care unit, each demonstrating their expertise. The professionals consulted each other on an equal level as they worked within their own professional boundaries.

On the ward there was less joined-up communication, and different professions worked independently. I reflected on this. Intensive care focuses on acute detail and the professionals contribute to understanding the case. On the ward, patients may be at different stages of recovery and have diverse needs. The opportunities to collaborate and interact can be disjointed, resulting in a task-based approach, so it can be difficult to construct a picture of each profession's contribution to holistic care. Through this experience I recognise that physiotherapists help with physical mobility rehabilitation and are vital in preventing chest infections by clearing the chest of secretions. Occupational therapists ensure that people are ready to manage independently at home. Doctors and nurses' roles overlap in that the doctors prescribe treatment based on nurses' observations. I think that interprofessional collaboration is based on professionals recognising each other's strengths and expertise and avoiding power issues.'

Activity 9.3 Reflection (page 164)

The articles required for this activity are:

- Farrell, G (2001) From tall poppies to squashed weeds. *Journal of Advanced Nursing*, 35: 26–33.
- Freshwater, D (2000) Crosscurrents against cultural narration in nursing. *Journal of Advanced Nursing*, 32(2): 481–4.
- Hutchinson, M, Vickers, M, Jackson, D and Wilkes, L (2006) Workplace bullying in nursing: towards a more critical organisational perspective. *Nursing Inquiry*, 13(2): 118–26.

Activity 9.5 Reflection on Mia's collaborative learning (page 167)

Mia broke corporate confidentiality by naming the healthcare trust that she worked in and the institution where she was studying. This meant that her work could, potentially, identify where any situation she was talking about was located. Some people call this the 'on the bus test'. Should the work be left in a public place, are there sufficient identifiers to locate where situations are happening? In terms of the consequences of breaching confidentiality, for Mia these would be greater (although these still depend on the seriousness of the breach), because she is a registered nurse and therefore accountable for her actions. The consequences for Josh, as a student, if he had followed the same actions as Mia, are less serious (although these still depend on the seriousness of the breach), because he has a responsibility for maintaining confidentiality, but is not yet a registered accountable practitioner. The best option is to leave any identifiers out of any account!

Activity 9.6 Reflection (page 169)

Although the content and structure of your reflection is likely to be unique to you, there are some common rules you might have followed. You might have plotted the reflective story as a sequence of scenes. If using poetic devices, you might have considered

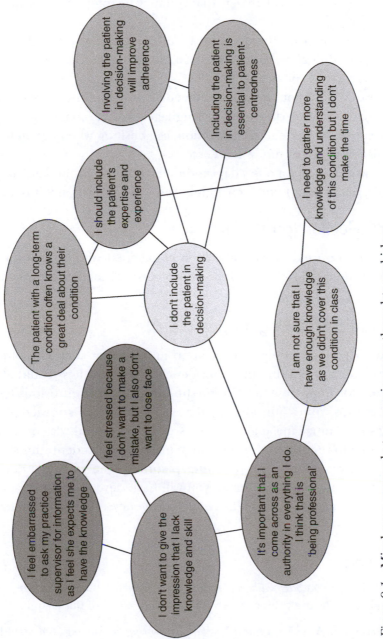

Figure 9.1 Mind map example to organise your thoughts and ideas

whether to use a chorus or rhyming mechanism to emphasise particular points. All of these considerations are important. When trying to write creatively, it is important take a few things into account:

- Use a quiet, comfortable location, with minimal distractions and where you feel safe enough to write without anxiety that you may be interrupted or questioned as to your activity.
- You need to organise your thoughts, ideas and/or emotions. It might help you to organise your thoughts if you construct a mind map that expresses your ideas (please see Figure 9.1 for an example).
- Read your work, slowly, out loud and then edit it by including extra or different punctuation, changing terminology or language, possibly changing the style from a passive to an active sentence construction, establishing whether you feel it should be in the present, past or future tense, etc.
- Leave your work to rest for a few days and then re-read it in the same way again and decide what (if anything) needs changing. You will know when it is ready.

Activity 9.7 Reflection (page 171)

The themes you identified might have been concerned with communication skills, decision-making and relationships with peers, practice colleagues, clients and tutors.

Activity 9.8 Critical thinking (pages 174–5)

You might have identified strengths in relation to particular skills and others that you wanted to improve. It is possible that confidence or assertiveness could also have featured as an area for improvement. You might know this from previous feedback and your own reflections. You might identify that you need more knowledge or practical skills. As a registered nurse this might involve some kind of study day or training, which you would be able to request from your line manager. As a student, this should inform your learning contract. Your reflection after planning your personal development is likely to be much more positive, because you will have developed some agency in your learning and development. (For the discussion on agency, return to Chapter 3.)

Further reading

Bolton, G (2014) *Reflective Practice: Writing and professional development*, 4th edn. Los Angeles, CA: Sage.
An in-depth guide to reflective writing, which is beyond the scope of this chapter.

Price, B and Harrington, A (2018) *Critical Thinking & Writing for Nursing Students*, 4th edn. London: Sage.
Good explanation and examples of how to write reflective essays applying critical thinking skills that map to the new NMC's *Standards of Proficiency for Registered Nurses* (NMC, 2018a).

Chapter 10　Using new media for reflecting

Chapter aims

After reading this chapter, you will be able to:

* identify different types of media that can be used for reflection;
* assess the advantages and avoid the pitfalls of using media for reflection;
* develop a reflective script for a media narrative;
* identify how you can contribute to others' reflective learning.

Introduction

Scenario 10.1: Sonia's reflective experience

Sonia has just started her paediatric nursing programme. One of the first tasks she is asked to do is to set up her electronic portfolio using different pages for different parts of her learning experience. Sonia is a bit concerned about completing this task because she has never used an e-portfolio tool before. However, after an introductory talk about how to get started from her course tutor, Julie, Sonia manages to set up her e-portfolio with named pages for her skills, personal development planning with actions, reflective diary and practice development.

Sonia starts to use her reflective journal to log her learning experiences of lectures. She mentions her clinical science tutor by name, saying how impressed she is with the resources he provides to the class. After sharing her e-portfolio for feedback on her writing, Julie comments that confidentiality needs to be maintained by not including people's names and that Sonia is ready to reflect on these experiences. Sonia goes back to her reflective journal and edits out the clinical science tutor's name and thinks about the 'so what' of her experience.

When Sonia starts her first placement she is very excited. She decides that it would be helpful for her learning to reflect on these early experiences. Each week she writes a reflective log about what she has learned in placement.

Remembering Julie's comment about maintaining confidentiality, Sonia ensures that she does not name any people, the placement or the organisation where it is located. Just before returning to university and submitting her e-portfolio, Sonia reflects on the sum total of her practice experiences by considering the question 'so what?' Julie places a further comment on Sonia's e-portfolio practice page affirming Sonia's reflective ability and her progression and learning from the feedback that she receives.

As technology progresses rapidly new media are constantly becoming available. This means that different opportunities for creative ways of reflecting are increasing. It is important in the digital age to become familiar with the diverse range of options available, to ensure not only that you make use of what is available, but also that you can engage with and teach others. Using e-technology in different ways will help prepare you for the ongoing electronic record changes and developments in practice. However, as highlighted in Scenario 10.1, media also pose potential problems that you need to guard against in order to protect those in your care and avoid misconduct resulting from not adhering to the NMC's Code (NMC, 2018b). The issue of confidentiality has always been an issue but use of media and the inability to specifically control information once it has been posted electronically (rather than using paper-based documentation) can result in unintended confidentiality breaches.

This chapter introduces some of the media that you might use in your reflective learning. It also highlights the opportunities and dangers posed by such media and identify ways that you can use media responsibly and professionally. The chapter also offers you an opportunity to develop a reflective script. The chapter concludes with how to translate this into a digital story.

Different types of media

Media refers to technological tools that have become available in recent years and that make connecting through the World Wide Web much easier. Technologies are continually being developed and the list of examples given below is clearly incomplete, but some of these technological tools are:

- social networking such as Facebook, YouTube, Instagram, etc.;
- instant messaging such as WhatsApp, Snapchat, WeChat, Twitter, Skype, Facebook Messenger, texting, etc.;
- e-mail;
- creative digital media, for example, image-sharing software such as Photo Story 3, Audacity, Windows Movie Maker, etc.

Ohler (2008) used the term 'new media' because it allowed for expansion and change in an evolving medium and still remains relevant. As has already been highlighted in Scenario 10.1, media offer different possibilities for reflection. One example of this is the e-portfolio which offers structure by providing templates to guide your information writing as well as the opportunity to collect feedback when they are shared. The information can be either kept private within the virtual learning environment or shared with others who need to be invited by you and accept the link you send them. Feedback is given via a comments button. This system clearly has advantages for the student, practice supervisor and personal tutor because, once all parties have been invited, progress can be followed, and communication and feedback provided in real time.

Your portfolio should include a section of reflective learning because this is a key aspect of the nursing code of conduct in terms of keeping your knowledge up to date (NMC, 2018b). The Nursing and Midwifery Council (NMC) expects all nurses to keep a portfolio and can call on this evidence at the point of registration and beyond (NMC, 2017). (See also *Successful Professional Portfolios for Nursing Students* (Reed, 2015) in this series.)

Social networking is useful for sharing ideas. It enables discussion of issues, sharing learning and following key experts through blogs. However, open sites such as Facebook and Twitter need to be used with caution, as discussed later in this chapter.

Creative media allow you to upload images and audio to create videos or digital stories offering the potential for more creative reflection. Examples of free download-able media programs that enable you to do this include Photo Story 3, Audacity and Windows Movie Maker, among others. These can be used to create media files from the images, sounds and narration that you input. It is important to maintain confidentiality from a different perspective when doing this because images can provide recognition of location and settings. Please be mindful that this consideration also applies to images of the university setting, clinical skills suite, simulation laboratories, etc.

Alternatively, you could use the narrated PowerPoint option in association with copyright-free images to create a Windows media video file. This harnesses different thought processes. For example, you might choose an image as a metaphor for what would require many words to explain. The viewer makes sense of the meaning framed by his or her own biographical experience (for more information on this, revisit Chapter 3). Creating stories requires discipline, structure, scripting, critical analysis and editing, which are also the skills needed for critical reflection. Please complete Activity 10.1 to consider how you might use media.

Activity 10.1   Reflection

- Using your knowledge of reflection from your reading so far make a list of the characteristics of any of the media tools mentioned above that would help you to reflect and why.
- In what ways do you think you might use the different media mentioned to reflect?
- Are there any other media, not mentioned, that you could use?

As this activity is based on your experience, there is no outline answer at the end of the chapter.

You might have considered how different forms of media allow you to express yourself differently in ways that are not yet fully formed. You might also have thought about how new media could enable you to interact with others to get feedback on your ideas, and to develop your reflective thinking and experience. However, although interaction can be an advantage, there are also some pitfalls to beware of. These are discussed in more detail in the next section.

Advantages and pitfalls of new media

Media, as has already been suggested, can enable dynamic articulation of reflections. This includes synchronous approaches such as social networking as well as asynchronous methods such as discussion boards and blogs. The advantages of these are that they bring nurses together in new ways and are not limited to locations, providing opportunities for development, making nurses' voices heard and sharing good practice (Falconer, 2011). For example, through talking to nurses from other countries, it is possible to compare and contrast different healthcare systems across the world and reflect on your own role at the same time. New media also make it easier to study at a distance and to keep in contact with developing ideas without having to sit in a classroom with others. This makes education programmes more accessible to a wider variety of people and provides opportunities for group work that would otherwise not be possible.

There are, however, also inherent risks. In discussions at the Royal College of Nursing (RCN, 2011) congress, David Jones highlighted that once information has been shared on a website it cannot be removed. Recognising that nurses use social networking sites, the NMC (2012) produced some guidance, noting that nurses and midwives will put their registration at risk and students may jeopardise their ability to join the register if they:

- share confidential information online;
- post inappropriate comments about staff or patients;
- use social networking sites to bully and intimidate colleagues;
- pursue personal relationships with patients and service users;
- distribute sexually explicit material;
- use social networking sites in a way that is unlawful.

The Nursing and Midwifery Council (NMC) advises that conduct in the real world and online should be viewed as one and the same, and conduct should always be in keeping with the standards of the NMC's Code (NMC, 2018b). You are invited to consider Scenario 10.2 and answer the questions in Activity 10.2.

Scenario 10.2: Stacey's image sharing experience

Stacey is a newly qualified, learning disability nurse. During her preparation programme Stacey kept in touch with her peers and university life via Facebook. Now she is qualified Stacey has updated her profile to reflect this. Stacey enjoys travelling and is a keen photographer. She enjoys sharing her images with her friends and usually uses Facebook to do so. She recently uploaded some images she had taken of tribal people on a holiday in Australia to Facebook and added some comments. Stacey is shocked when she is called to see her manager because a complaint had been made about how she was representing the equality and diversity policy of her organisation.

Our interpretation of images is subjective and can result in unintended consequences. Stacey may have had very different ideas about the purpose of her images to those of other viewers. The fact that she has listed her occupation on her profile may further influence viewers' ideas about what she might be trying to say through posting her images. The narrative of images is a strong focus of media offering creative potential but, as Stacey's experience highlights, there are also responsibilities to consider.

The RCN (2009) has produced legal advice on using the internet. This emphasises the importance of reading and adhering to the information technology (IT) policy of the organisation you are in and ensuring that you uphold the reputation of both your profession and the organisation. For the qualified practitioner, this means ensuring that personal behaviour does not compromise professional standing. For the student nurse this would mean the organisations within which your preparation programme and your placements are located. The RCN (2009, p2) recommends that you:

- avoid any identification of your employer;
- under no circumstances identify patients in your care or post information that might lead to the identification of a patient;
- do not air grievances where others might read them;
- do not make disparaging remarks about an employer, colleagues or clients.

Most of this is straightforward advice to follow, but there are times when boundaries blur and it can be difficult to remember who you are professionally. Consider Scenario 10.3 and complete Activity 10.2 to clarify what you think you would do.

Scenario 10.3: Alistair's social networking experience

Alistair was working in the community on placement with practice nurses at a GP surgery. He enjoyed this placement because of the diversity of the work and the people with whom he came into contact. He became very friendly with his practice supervisor, Colin. Alistair asked Colin if he would be interested in becoming a friend on his social networking site. Colin agreed and told Alistair to send him an invitation. That evening Alistair was on the site and sent Colin an invitation to become a friend. In his invitation Alistair said that he very much enjoyed working with Colin at the GP surgery. Colin accepted the invitation and he and Alistair have been swapping messages about their interests outside work. There are some issues that Alistair wants to learn more about in relation to his placement, but he does not discuss these on the social networking site because this would not be appropriate. He catches up with Colin at work about them instead. At the end of his placement Alistair asks Colin to keep in touch, which he agrees to do.

Activity 10.2   Reflection

After reading Scenario 10.2 about Stacey's experience and Scenario 10.3 about Alistair and Colin, answer the following questions:

- What should Stacey have thought about before uploading her photos and comments?
- What are the main issues in the case study concerning Alistair and Colin?
- What might be the outcomes for Stacey, Alistair and Colin?
- What might you do differently?

There are outline answers to these questions at the end of the chapter.

The above activity has offered you the opportunity to think about some of the challenges involved in separating professional and private life, and keeping appropriate boundaries, particularly when you feel that people are friends. Reflecting on such experiences is important for developing and maintaining professional behaviour. Your professional integrity is essential to becoming registered or keeping your registration if you are a registered practitioner. We continue to consider positive ways in which media can be used for reflection by exploring how to develop stories.

Developing a reflective story using new media

Storytelling has been a traditional part of human communication for centuries and stories are a useful tool for developing understanding (Davidhizar and Lonser, 2003). Considering a significant issue and creating the story that surrounds it helps to clarify your thinking and reasoning, and to reflect differently than is possible in a written assignment (Matthews-DeNatale, 2008). According to Boase (2008, p9), developing reflective stories using new media enables you to:

- promote deep reflection, review, analysis and ordering of information (e.g. a project, a topic, an experience);
- value emotional/personal input;
- make sense of experience;
- encourage cooperative activity;
- create powerful end-products that can have a transformative effect on maker and viewer alike;
- develop capacity for self-review;
- build confidence.

The process of creating the story helps to make it an embodied experience, which allows you to visualise and relive the situation, and it is important for deepening your understanding and learning. What is meant by embodiment is that the experience is lived and owned by you as the person reflecting, and unconscious aspects are brought to light. Our experiences are informed by the 'appearance, disappearance and reappearance of events and people making our world seem familiar' (Horsdal, 2012, p10). However, we cannot perceive these influences unless we can see the whole story. To do this you need first to develop a script, an example of which can be seen below.

A script about person-centred care

'Where's Mike?' asked the menacing-looking individual at the desk. Maggie glanced at me nervously. 'Room 9', I calmly replied. He walked up the corridor and disappeared into Mike's room. Mike had been transferred to the limb surgery unit following a motorcycle accident. He had been filtering to go off a roundabout and had been crushed by a lorry. His lower leg was damaged beyond repair and had to be amputated. Mike was struggling to come to terms with his injury, often becoming angry and resentful. The man visiting him was clearly a motorcyclist too.

This is my first qualified nurse post and I am still getting used to it. I am learning how to dress stump wounds and bandage them correctly. What I am finding harder, though, is learning how to connect with the wounded person. I come from a background where people are valued as individuals and I want to use those values in my nursing. The problem is, how do I work with Mike in a way that is meaningful for him and values his individuality?

We start to chat. Mike says that he finds the limb surgery unit boring because there is nothing for him to do. I ask him what he normally does. He says that he works on art designs for motorcycles. He has a website where he showcases his work, and people contact him or they approach him at the events he attends. He doesn't want to miss the motorcycle show at the end of the month. He is worried that his business will suffer. I talk to the occupational therapist and ask her to source some art materials for Mike. Mike starts to use these to create design ideas and appears more purposeful. I also talk to the physiotherapist about his objective of getting to the motorcycle show. The physiotherapist tailors Mike's exercise regime to include walking on uneven terrain.

At the end of the month Mike's friend, who no longer appears to be menacing as we have come to know him better, takes Mike to the motorcycle show. I think I will ask Mike if he is willing to share his experiences and recovery with others as we do get several biker patients.

Read Scenario 10.4 and then complete Activity 10.3.

Scenario 10.4: Naeve's critical incident experience

Naeve was working in a mental health secure unit placement. She was in the third year of her mental health nursing programme, and was due to qualify in three months. She had finished a stretch of duties and, on one of her days off, decided to reflect on a particular issue that had given her work satisfaction. The unit had some patients with complex problems. One of these was Jeff, who had been sectioned and admitted after smashing up the family home and having a stand-off with the police. He had been off work with severe stress preceding this event. His family had found the experience of his outburst extremely traumatic and were reluctant to visit him. He had a sister who lived two hours' travelling time away. Naeve could see that Jeff was withdrawn and did not speak much. Each day that she was on shift she spent some time sitting with him, trying to draw him out. By the second week he was starting to mumble some responses. By the third week Naeve managed to coax Jeff to come downstairs for his lunch. His sister had been enquiring after Jeff regularly. In that third week Naeve asked Jeff if he wanted to see his sister and he agreed. Jeff asked for Naeve to be present when they met.

Jeff's sister Miriam met him in the common room. At first everything appeared to be going well, but then Jeff lost his temper when Miriam asked him where he would go on leaving the unit because he could not go back home. Naeve ushered Miriam out of the room and returned to Jeff. Although she felt anxious inside, Naeve was able to maintain a calm exterior, which gradually helped Jeff to calm down. Naeve's practice supervisor, Andrew, had been observing her communication interactions during this interaction and was very impressed with Naeve's handling of this volatile situation. Andrew gave Naeve a glowing report before she left this placement.

Naeve used a private blog to reflect on the incident and her overall feelings about the placement over the last few weeks. She felt she had made some real progress in her communication and interaction with Jeff. She found this satisfying because it appeared to affirm her communication ability. When Jeff had become agitated and angry in his interaction with his sister, Naeve had reacted quickly to remove Miriam from danger and calm the situation, despite feeling a bit fearful herself. She knew that this was part of what she would need to do as a mental health nurse, and was pleased that the way in which she had handled the critical incident had been affirmed by her practice supervisor. When she considered what she might have done differently she thought about whether she should have called for help or sent Miriam to get help when she left the room. The reason she had not done this was because she felt confident in her own abilities and the therapeutic relationship she had established with Jeff. Naeve thought that the worst that could have happened was that Jeff might have struck her, but as she had had training in breakaway techniques she felt able to take care of herself to get away if necessary, but she preferred to use communication to resolve the situation. The incident had increased her confidence in being able to manage different situations effectively and she felt more prepared for qualifying in the next few months.

Activity 10.3   Reflection

- Use the scenario above to develop a story script about the incident and Naeve's reflection on it.
- Now try to write a story script for a critical incident you have experienced and your reflection on it.

There is an outline answer to part of this activity at the end of the chapter.

Writing an event as a script helps you to deconstruct and examine different elements before reassembling them in a cohesive whole. A script normally starts with a significant event that engages the reader's attention from the start and has an unfolding plot that connects different aspects in a whole (Boase, 2008). This requires critical awareness in knowing what to select and what to leave out and how to substantiate important points. The script should be approximately 200–300 words in length (Matthews-DeNatale, 2008). As stated by Boase (2008, p10), the skills involved in creating a story using new media include:

- narrative generation;
- reflection;
- analysis of material;
- analysis of self in relation to material;
- organising and sorting information for use;
- use of personal and technological/technical skills.

The first step is to match the script with appropriate images. To do this you will need to access the software that you intend to use and create a storyboard (this can be a series of boxes that link the plot of the script with numbered images). This allows you to place your chosen images on an editing line similar to a film strip. Images can be sourced from your own photographs, from photo-share sites such as **www.flickr.com** and from hand drawings. It is important to make sure that you check and follow copyright rules for any shared images and that you gain consent for any personal photos involving other people. The next step is to convert the script into an audio file using an appropriate audio editing tool. An example is Audacity, which records you narrating the script. Or, if you are planning to use PowerPoint, you could use the recording element to narrate to PowerPoint. Try to do this in as natural a way as possible in a quiet space, as if you were talking to someone. If using PowerPoint, make sure that you wait for any transitions to have completed to avoid words being cut off. This is the first step to converting the script into a digital story. Once you have matched your audio with the images, you can add titles and save your project. At this stage you should still be able to edit it. You are now ready to review your project file and reflect on whether the story portrays what you intended. It is also helpful at this stage to get other people's feedback, because then you can make editing changes before completing the final story package. Complete Activity 10.4 to see what you can produce.

Activity 10.4   Reflection

(Note: You will need a headset with a microphone for this activity.)

Download Photo Story 3 from **http://microsoft-photo-story.en.softonic.com** on to your computer:

- Find a photo that holds a special meaning for you.
- Think about the memories that are triggered by the photo and write a story script about these using the guidance previously given.
- Translate this script into a digital story using the new media software and following the prompts, as suggested above.
- Review your digital story and the processes used to create it and reflect on what you have learned.

As this activity is based on your own experiences, there is no outline answer at the end of the chapter.

We now proceed to explore how sharing stories that have been created using media can contribute to the reflective learning of others.

Contributing to the reflective learning of others

Sharing your development of the digital story with peers and teachers not only helps you to increase the quality of the final product, but also contributes to the reflective learning of others as they explore the meaning that they make from viewing your story. It is therefore useful to share your practice with others in order to collaborate in reflecting. As technology progresses, more advanced media are increasingly being used within nursing programmes to bring the service-user voice to the fore and to develop learning in more engaging ways. Examples that are used can be found on the Patient Voices website at **www.patientvoices.org.uk.** It is interesting to view different stories and share your reflections on them.

Chapter summary

This chapter has explored how to use media to develop reflection in different ways. Some of the advantages and pitfalls have been highlighted to help you use these new

(Continued)

(Continued)

opportunities constructively, and guard against creating problems for yourself that could affect you professionally and jeopardise your registration. The activities have offered you opportunities to develop your own digital story to reflect on. In the process you will have developed and practised media skills that you can take forward in your own learning and that you can use to contribute to the reflections of others.

Activities and scenarios: Brief outline answers

Activity 10.2 Reflection on Stacey's image-sharing experience and Alistair's social networking experience (page 189)

The main issues that arise in Scenario 10.2 are:

- Stacey has identified that she is a qualified children's nurse and therefore accountable for her actions;
- she is not properly adhering to her organisation's equality and diversity policy or the NMC's code.

In Scenario 10.3, involving Alistair and Colin, issues arise through:

- the blurring of Alistair's and Colin's professional and private lives as evidenced in their social networking communication;
- Alistair's mention in his invitation that they both work in a GP surgery.

The potential outcomes for Stacey are that she may receive a warning, which will be kept on her file because she is accountable for her actions. For Alistair, any feedback that Colin gives him as his practice supervisor may be viewed through the lens of social networking and, potentially, not be taken seriously. The potential outcomes for Colin are that he is accountable for his actions and could be putting his registration at risk. By blurring the boundary between his professional role as practice supervisor and communicating socially with Alistair online, Colin cannot guarantee what Alistair might say. Other people could access the posts and that could have professional repercussions. As a student, you might think that it is innocent to develop a friendship with someone. However, as a practice supervisor or assessor, it is inappropriate to be overly friendly with a student you supervise or assess. Social networking with someone while you are also supporting them in a professional capacity is a potential risk to your registration. Reflecting on this, it would be beneficial for both parties to inform yourselves about policies and guidance on using media within the organisation and from a regulation perspective. The NMC's Code, in the section *Promote professionalism and trust* (item 20.3), explicitly identifies this and refers the reader to their online guidance (**www.nmc-uk.org/guidance**). Reading through this section, you will note that other items (20.5–20.8) are also relevant to these scenarios. Other aspects of the NMC's

Code (NMC, 2018b) about confidentiality and protecting personal rights are also applicable and it is strongly recommended that in addition you consider Scenarios 10.2 and 10.3 from these broader perspectives of professional practice.

Activity 10.3 Reflection on Naeve's critical incident experience (page 192)

The script might go as follows:

'Get out you stupid woman', he shouted, raising his fist at his sister. I hurriedly ushered her out of the room and then went back to try to calm him down. He had come to the unit after smashing up his home and threatening the police and his family. For the last three weeks I have been trying to build up a therapeutic relationship with him to get him to communicate and come out of himself more. I had not intended for him to react like this, though, when I told his sister he was ready to see her. I should be scared, but I feel calm. He is out of control, but I feel in control of the situation. The preparation I have had has, I think, helped me feel this way. What would I do if he hits me? Others might say, 'It is your own fault because you did not ask for help.' I would have to rethink my strategy. But for now, things are calming down. I go home feeling great after the glowing report from my practice supervisor. My communication strategies have been rewarded and affirmed by the patient calming down and my practice supervisor praising my handling of the situation. I feel ready to progress towards being a qualified nurse.

Further reading

Nursing and Midwifery Council (NMC) (2012) *Social Networking Sites*. Available at: www.nmc-uk.org/Nurses-and-midwives/Advice-by-topic/A/Advice/Social-networking-sites

Reed, S (2015) *Successful Professional Portfolios for Nursing Students*, 2nd edn. London: Sage.

Royal College of Nursing (RCN) (2009) *Legal Advice for RCN Members Using the Internet*. London: RCN. Available at: www.rcn.org.uk/data/assets/pdf_file/0008/272195/003557.pdf

Useful websites

http://digitalstorytelling.coe.uh.edu

This website offers a tutorial and a range of guidance on creating your own digital story. You are encouraged to explore the whole website to view what it has to offer in terms of reflection examples.

www.nmc-uk.org

The Nursing and Midwifery Council's website provides information on the latest regulations and what nurses and midwives need to do to adhere to them.

www.patientvoices.org.uk

This website offers a range of stories involving patients and nurses in diverse settings and situations. These provide useful examples for this genre of storytelling.

www.rcn.org.uk

The Royal College of Nursing's website offers advice and guidance on issues relating to nursing. It also has discussion forums where nurses can share practice.

Chapter 11 Critical reflection

Chapter aims

After reading this chapter you will be able to:

- critically examine personal contributions and those of others within practical and psychological considerations;
- explore the limits of your understanding;
- assess sources of evidence within any situation;
- identify the coming together of new ideas.

Introduction

Scenario 11.1: Meg gives first aid

Meg was in the third year of her nursing programme. On her way home from an early shift, she stopped at the supermarket. As Meg rounded the corner to the dairy aisle, she came across a man on the floor. Meg placed him in the recovery position and observed that he appeared stiff and rigid and was *cyanosed*. Meg recognised this as the *tonic* phase of an *epileptic fit* and cleared a space around him so that, as the *clonic* phase of jerking started, he would not injure himself. Meg continued to monitor that he started breathing again as the tonic phase gave way to the clonic phase. At this point someone came up to Meg and told her he was a first aider and that she should put something between the man's teeth to stop him biting his tongue. Meg was not sure whether this was right and decided not to follow the advice. The store staff had called an ambulance and, when the paramedics arrived, Meg told them what she had done and then completed her shopping and went home.

When she got home, Meg was surprised to find she was rather shaken by the event. She tried to analyse what had happened and why she was feeling this way. She realised that her shakiness was a reaction to the adrenaline rush she had experienced on finding the man collapsed on the floor. Although this had helped to focus her mind on what was important, it also had the physiological consequences that she was now experiencing.

Meg critically reflected on her actions. Looking back, she thought that perhaps she should have checked the man for other signs, such as looking at his pupils and checking for any injury, because there are several reasons why someone might be fitting. She was satisfied to have put the man in the recovery position so quickly and to have protected his airway. Meg thought about what the person claiming to be a first aider had said about putting something between the man's teeth. As she still was not sure, she decided to check what her nursing literature recommended and found that this action was positively discouraged. Meg was glad she had not listened, but also thought critically about what had led her to this decision. Turning someone into the recovery position was a way to ensure the tongue did not fall back and block the airway, and therefore pushing something into the mouth at the same time was likely to achieve the opposite effect and potentially force the tongue backwards. Meg had instinctively grasped the danger and avoided it. However, she realised that, had she been in the first year of her preparation programme, she might have listened, assuming that the man claiming to be a first aider was correct. This led her to reflect on how you could not know the experience, qualifications and knowledge of anyone who stops to help in an emergency. It was important in every situation to work within her own competence and knowledge levels so as not to do harm. Meg was glad that she had waited for the ambulance staff to help instead. She decided that she would do a more thorough initial assessment in future to ensure that she did not miss anything important.

Becoming a professional is about developing criticality to analyse and identify significant priorities and potential solutions. As you progress through your programme you will develop critical skills from first observations to more complex decision-making. In Meg's case she used her initial observations to make decisions about the priorities – the person's airway. Critical reflection enabled her to recognise limitations in her knowledge and ways to remedy these.

This chapter emphasises the importance of critical reflection and its relevance to the developing skill of criticality. It also offers you opportunities to engage in critical reflection through different activities and scenarios. How new ideas come together as the final part of an analytical process are considered at the end.

Critically examining personal contributions and those of others

Critical reflection differs from other forms of reflection in that it examines and questions all the factors involved in a situation from a critical perspective, which makes the familiar unfamiliar. This means looking at routine situations as if they were new to find out what might be seen differently. This requires disciplined thought to achieve the depth of analysis required. Such a questioning approach is also directed at personal actions to investigate motives, assumptions and decision-making, and what you were really thinking. The frameworks offered in Chapter 4 provide encompassing structures that can be used to direct a critical approach. Critical reflection, used with critical incident analysis such as reviewing and analysing situations, is important for learning and can help to build case studies from which to learn (Rolfe, 2011). Activity 11.1 can help you to begin critical incident analysis and develop your learning by examining your contributions and those of others to learn from them.

Activity 11.1   Critical thinking

Critical incident analysis is a form of debrief that looks back at situations to consider what needs to be learned. Review what you have done, or been involved with, in the last few weeks and choose an incident to review. Write a detailed account of the event, including your own and others' actions. Now consider the following questions:

- Why is this situation significant for you?
- How did it affect you?

(Continued)

(Continued)

- How did you feel about it?
- What was satisfying about the situation?
- What was concerning about the situation?
- What might you have done differently?
- Was there any additional knowledge that you needed?
- Where might you go to find it?
- What have you learned?
- How will you take this learning forward?

There are outline answers to this activity at the end of the chapter.

Having reviewed your incident, you might like to go further by considering who was responsible and who was accountable in the situation, and any implications in terms of significance, concerns and potential consequences. How does this inform your thinking about being a nurse?

As this is based on your own experiences, there is no outline answer at the end of the chapter.

Examining situations in this systematic way may be time-consuming, but they ensure that situations and cases are *studied* for what can be learned and what can be taken forward as situational and experiential evidence. Connecting this with other forms of knowledge adds to the evidence base. It can be helpful to write a pen portrait of the situation. Writing a pen portrait enables you to bring elements together that are relevant to the situation and the individuals involved, thus providing a complete picture and building on the storytelling we discussed in Chapter 10. A pen portrait should address the following:

- the history and context of the situation;
- own and others' interpretations and analysis of what was happening;
- own use of knowledge;
- own and others' actions and consequences of those actions;
- insights arising from reflection;
- link of insights to evidence base.

Pen portrait example

I am working on a care for older people ward. A woman – Mavis – was admitted last week after a fall. Her neighbours had found her on the floor unable to get up. At first it was assumed that Mavis had broken her ankle because her foot was so painful. Further

(Continued)

(Continued)

investigation revealed she had cellulitis requiring antibiotics. Mavis also has diabetes and her blood count showed severe iron deficiency anaemia. At handover Mavis was presented as being uncooperative with treatment by refusing analgesia and physiotherapy attempts at rehabilitation. She would lie on the bed with her eyes closed. The bed manager is keen that discharge planning should progress.

I can see that Mavis is exhausted. Talking with her has identified that maintaining her autonomy is important to her. Colleagues have told me they think Mavis is not looking after herself properly and therefore not coping on her own. My knowledge of psychology suggests that Mavis is reacting to threats to her autonomy. Working with her in a more person-centred way may achieve better results.

I have started by asking Mavis what she wants, how she would like to achieve it and if she wants us to help in any way. Mavis seems more alert when I do this. Some colleagues think I am wasting time and I have noticed that Mavis is less co-operative with them.

Reflecting on Mavis's situation I think the sudden loss of her autonomy has caused upset and resistance. If I were in her shoes, I would probably also feel angry to not be consulted about what was happening to me. Consultation seems to be the key point here. Although dignity and respect are part of professional codes, it seems that subjective judgements are still made about people. It might be useful to have a lunchtime discussion about care and compassion and the 6 Cs.

Healthcare needs to be organised around individuals not processes, as appears to be happening here. Applying the principles of person-centred care empowers individuals to make choices for themselves and become partners in their care, thereby preparing them to continue in their own environments. In the example above, dignity and respect are mentioned as being part of the Nursing and Midwifery Council's (NMC's) Code (NMC, 2018b). It is important, however, not to simply name these without exploring them in more detail. Please take time to explore the Code and identify which elements would be relevant to Mavis's situation.

Critical incident analysis may be applied to positive and negative situations. Consider the following case study to see how this might be done.

Case study: Elimu's compliment

Elimu was in the final year of his nurse preparation programme and working on a stroke unit. This was an extended placement, enabling Elimu to really get to know the patients and staff and feel a part of the team. Elimu was putting the management principles that he was learning on his nursing programme into practice. During a particularly busy shift, one of the patients suffered a cardiac arrest. Elimu was close by and called for help and then calmly initiated the resuscitation protocol. At the end of the shift his practice supervisor complimented Elimu on his swift actions, calm manner and correct responses.

Elimu thought about this critically on his way home, deconstructing the chain of events and reviewing his actions. He considered whether there had been any warning signs that perhaps he might have missed that the patient was about to arrest, but the nursing observations he had recorded earlier had not changed. Elimu felt that he had responded as quickly as was possible and his response was linked to good visual observation of his patients. He had called for help so that the resuscitation team could be alerted, and other staff would join him. This had resulted in someone bringing the necessary equipment. In the meantime, Elimu had been able to commence cardiopulmonary resuscitation because he had learned how to do this in class. He analysed how this felt different from practising on the simulation mannequin. He needed to concentrate on the amount of force he used in order to maintain consistency. It was also much more tiring than he had anticipated, confirming another reason to seek help.

As part of his management course Elimu had discussed different types of leadership and delegation in a variety of situations, and this knowledge helped him to respond calmly and effectively. However, Elimu recognised that his knowledge of the different drugs that the team used when they arrived was limited. He decided that learning these was something he would take forward from the situation. However, his practice supervisor's compliment had affirmed his actions and so he recognised that these were appropriate to the situation.

The case study identifies the importance of the team in responding to situations and for peer feedback. Interpersonal relationships are important for team building and peer support, and can be used for critically examining personal contributions and those of others. Anyone, including the student nurse, relies on peers when entering new clinical environments (Petty, 2014). Peer support also involves offering constructive feedback to develop practice. This can be difficult, because it is easy to become critical rather than being critically constructive.

Trust needs to be developed to facilitate learning critically. Building trust involves three arenas comprising risk, example and consistency (Curzon-Hobson, 2002). Reflection and open dialogue are helpful to support trust in sensitive circumstances because students can find integrating into an unknown environment intimidating, whether this is a programme, a new module, or a new placement area in practice (Dix and Hughes, 2004). Consider Scenario 11.2 and reflect critically on integrating new staff into a team.

> ## Scenario 11.2: Integrating a new member of staff
>
> A new member of staff recently joined the team. The new member of staff requires constant attention and support, making it difficult for me to get on with my job. I have allocated time to catch up, but she still constantly interrupts me for guidance, instead of problem-solving for herself. She is also given exceptional leeway as to flexible working time to accommodate her childcare, which is now putting extra pressure on the rest of us because we have to manage after she has left early.

Activity 11.2   Critical reflection

After critically reflecting on this scenario:

- What do you think are the main reflective points from the perspectives of both the experienced practitioner and the new member of staff?
- What potential learning points have you identified and how might these be applied in practice?

There are outline answers to these questions at the end of the chapter.

The ability to critically examine personal contributions in relationship with others opens a different point of view that is more empathetic and therefore supportive of staff relationships. This leads to a positive atmosphere, where it is possible to offer constructive criticism that does not offend people, but from which they learn the limits of their understanding. Mutual understanding and respect allows trust to develop and forms the foundation of healthy team relationships.

Exploring the limits of understanding

Critically reflecting on the limits of your understanding is important for both the novice and experienced practitioner and is enshrined within the NMC's Code (NMC, 2018b). Even if you were previously competent in a skill or knowledgeable in a particular area, you can become unskilled over time, or things could change, meaning that your knowledge and understanding are not up to date. Healthcare is constantly evolving so that things change, and new learning is required to maintain your skill set and ensure that you stay abreast of new developments. A critical, reflective stance towards your practice will enable you to identify deficits in your knowledge and skill base, and recognise the limits of your understanding. In Chapter 9, we saw that writing reflections facilitates your analysis of experiences, stimulates new ideas and increases awareness of new learning which could, otherwise, remain invisible (Chirema, 2007). To do this involves critically reviewing daily experience and analysing it, raising awareness of how you are learning and what new knowledge you are developing. Tappen et al. (2010) suggest that critical thinking requires individuals to continually examine their thinking processes, looking for gaps and identifying supporting evidence and potential consequences of their decisions for others and themselves.

For example, when thinking about why you react in particular ways to certain situations, you may impose a psychological reasoning process and compare your responses with those set within the criteria. You may then question the assumptions you have used and assess your thinking in relation to these. Determining strengths, limitations and opportunities involves imagining the possible consequences of thinking in this way. Consider the next case study to identify how thinking critically can be a starting point for critical reflection.

Case study: Rob's dyslexia

Rob was in the first year of his nursing programme. He had not had an easy time learning at school and found the programme was becoming difficult because he had to complete several written assignments. Rob decided to reflect critically on the problems with his learning and explore the options available to him.

Rob considered the problems he had with reading and writing, and how he would never have an easy time in formal learning. He realised that he was not able to retain information in the same way that others could when he related his abilities to the graduate skills that were expected of him. Rob considered that he was good at creative problem-solving and working with people, but he was concerned that he would not be able to function at the same level as other practitioners. Rob realised that, to move forward, he had to first overcome his fear.

When reflecting critically, Rob realised that the way that he saw things differently was a positive thing because he could see alternative solutions that others could not. Rob also saw that he needed structure to help him understand how to learn new concepts, and this was why he found self-directed study and activities hard. Rob noted that he wrote himself notes and scribbles as a way of reinforcing particular points. Handouts did not help him as he focused more on people talking.

Rob spoke to the study support department at his university. He also asked his tutors whether he could audio-record their teaching. This strategy meant that he could write down what was important when listening in class and when listening to the recording later. In this way he was able to access the information better. It also gave him a better idea of what to write about in his assignments as well as a chance to be reflective.

The case study may have helped you to identify that limits to understanding may also relate to your ability to engage with study. This is an important area to explore for you to be able to reflectively find strategies that work for you. Undertaking Activity 11.3 can help you to identify limits to your understanding and ways to address these.

Activity 11.3   Reflection

Think about a recent situation where you were not sure what to do. Consider the following questions and try to structure your reflection using one of the reflective models discussed in Chapter 4.

- What alerted you to the uncertainty?
- What did you know?
- What did you not know?
- What were the consequences?
- What might have been the consequences if you had known?
- What can you do about this?
- What learning do you take from this situation?

As this activity is based on your own experiences, there is no outline answer at the end of the chapter.

You may have identified that there are specific areas that you need to learn more about, or that there are some skills that you need to develop or refresh. This is part of being a reflective practitioner and will remain core to your professional practice throughout your career. Consider Scenario 11.3 about how exploring limits to knowledge can be an important safety issue.

Scenario 11.3: Fajid's understanding of young carers

Fajid was in the first year of his children's nursing programme. He was on his third placement, which was with the school nurses. His practice supervisor, Simon, involved Fajid in *health promotion* activities, working with schools on their healthy eating strategies. He was also involved in vaccination sessions. Part of the school nurse's role was to support pupils who had behavioural problems and follow up absenteeism. Simon was currently working with Kate who was a young carer for her mum. Simon and Fajid visited her at home to assess the situation and find ways to empower Kate. Fajid discussed Kate's situation when he and Simon left the house. He wondered why Kate, who was only 14 years old, was left caring for her mother.

Activity 11.4   Reflection

- What are the limits to Fajid's understanding in this scenario? What might be the consequences for Kate, her mum and Fajid?

There is an outline answer to this question at the end of the chapter.

In Scenario 11.3, Simon helped Fajid's learning by asking him to reflect critically on his actions, the potential consequences of his actions and the breadth of the nurse's professional role. Our ability to identify the sources of evidence used and to rectify deficits are important in maintaining safe practice. We can now critically assess the sources of evidence in a given situation.

Assessing sources of evidence within the situation

It is necessary for novice and experienced practitioners to reflect critically on the evidence base of their actions to provide good-quality patient care and identify their learning needs, and is an important part of developing your practice at any stage. This means examining the sources of evidence used when planning patient care and making decisions. Activity 11.5 can help you consider the sources of evidence used in a situation.

Activity 11.5   Critical thinking

Think of a situation from your experience in practice. Examine the sources of evidence supporting your interpretations and your decision-making, using the following questions:

- How did you assess the situation?
- What was your assessment based on?
- How did you know what to base it on?
- Was your interpretation correct?
- What confirmed that it was correct?
- If it was not correct, what evidence did you have that it was not correct?
- What did you base your subsequent decision on?
- How did you know it was the right decision?

As this activity is based on your personal experiences, there is an outline answer to only part of this activity at the end of the chapter.

A useful way of evaluating results from the activity above is to use a practice development tool called Claims, Concerns and Issues (McCormack et al., 2004, p95; Manley et al., 2014, p13). Claims are favourable assertions about things, Concerns are unfavourable assertions and Issues are questions you might reasonably ask about implementation. Use these terms as headings for three columns and list all your assertions and questions under the appropriate heading. Finally, think about using active questions that will help you to turn issues into positive results. They are a useful guide to ongoing critical reflection.

Confidence to communicate the evidence base for your actions is often subject to the culture in the workplace or the classroom. Lack of managerial or tutor support in situations can reduce co-operation and promote organisational friction. It is important to critically analyse factors such as leadership and your responses to it in order to identify facilitative and hindering factors that might also affect situations and decision-making.

Scenario 11.4: Arunda's experience of dealing with pressure

Arunda was a student in the second year of her nursing programme. She was working in an *endoscopy* suite. The unit was short staffed and had many complex patients to deal with. Although Arunda was supposed to be supernumerary, she had to work as a regular member of staff to help them deal with the complex patients. One in particular caused her concern. The patient was an alcoholic and attended for an *oesophageal gastroduodenoscopy* (*OGD*) procedure. The results showed that he had oesophageal varices, which are enlarged veins at the base of the oesophagus. Arunda was responsible for monitoring his vital signs. Arunda alerted the team that the vital signs were changing, and she thought that he had started to bleed. Stabilising the patient took some time. Afterwards Arunda helped to clean and decontaminate the equipment. Arunda and the team went off duty late. Just before they were leaving the manager praised Arunda, telling her she had done a good job. The following week Arunda asked her practice supervisor if she could take back some of the time she had used staying behind to help with the emergency. She wanted to see her daughter's school play. The manager was on holiday at the time and Arunda's practice supervisor (who had not been present at the emergency) refused, saying Arunda still had a lot to learn in her last week. Arunda met with her university link tutor who asked her how her placement had been. Arunda said it had been tough, but she had learned a lot.

Activity 11.6   Reflection

- What sources of evidence might Arunda use to evaluate her learning?
- What sources of evidence was the manager using to evaluate Arunda's learning?

- What sources of evidence was the practice supervisor using to evaluate Arunda's learning?

There are outline answers to these questions at the end of the chapter.

When interpretations are not checked for their validity it is possible for our fears and anxieties to become projected on to another person or situation, and for us to interact with that person or situation as if they meant us harm. Reading the points of guidance suggested at the end of this chapter about Scenario 11.4, you will notice that the situation can be interpreted in different ways depending on your role, responsibility and experience. Here, critical reflection helps us make sense of the evidence supporting the validity of our interpretations and how ideas fit together.

Identifying the coming together of new ideas

Critical reflection offers you psychological space to connect with your ideas and those of others, as well as the mental focus to do so. Your ideas and knowledge may be broad, but you also need to be open to consider challenging ideas in order to progress. This means drawing together ideas of process, building relationships, caring and ethical behaviours to inform the practice of nursing. Nursing knowledge is interconnected, emerging as a discipline in its own right while, as practitioners, you construct your ideas and contribute to this body of nursing knowledge. This role of authorship promotes reflexive dialogue with the ideas obtained from external sources as you progress through your nursing career. This process allows you to develop agency because you also focus on personal development and practice innovation.

We could argue that lack of feedback reduces the possibility of developing ideas. Therefore, discussing your reflections critically with someone is an important component of bringing new ideas together. During your nursing programme you will need the support of peers, practice supervisors, lecturers and clinical colleagues to allow you to develop new ideas of how to act and think as a professional. Even as experienced practitioners, we need the support of colleagues to challenge and discuss our practice in positive ways because this will stimulate creativity, criticality and imagination. Through this interaction we become more proactive in looking for ideas and answers, rather than simply accepting them and maintaining a status quo. These important steps build curiosity, imagination and learning that is life-long and critical.

To illustrate this, Figure 11.1 shows how ideas from the different ways of reflecting that have been discussed throughout this book are brought together. The outer world encompasses learning that is generated by political systems, organisational structures and scientific enquiry, and is represented by codified knowledge. This learning can be associated with the guidance that is offered, to be internally considered. For example, your practice supervisors and lecturers might identify what you need to learn, give you information and direct you to complete learning tasks. If you are an experienced practitioner you may be engaging with continuing professional development (CPD) courses or mandatory training, both of which may be prescribed by the employer or registering body. However, only you can make sense of what things mean to you and what you are taking forward through your 'inner world consideration'.

Political, cognitive, scientific and professional ideas are usually consistent with outer world experiences that intrude on the personal world, where they are met by inner world sense making. The interface between your outer and inner world experience is fluid in that it allows experiences and learning to interact. The inner world encompasses critical learning that helps to internalise experiences and may also be influential in shaping new ones, for example, in the level of self-confidence a person has or their self-esteem. This inner world includes biographical, personal and emotional dimensions, and reflexive, imaginative and creative responses to these dimensions. It is also where your values are embedded. These might relate to the continuous internal dialogue that you have with yourself in response to what is happening externally – namely, your emotional life, which influences your reactions, and maybe biographical memories, which are a part of your sense making as discussed in Chapter 3.

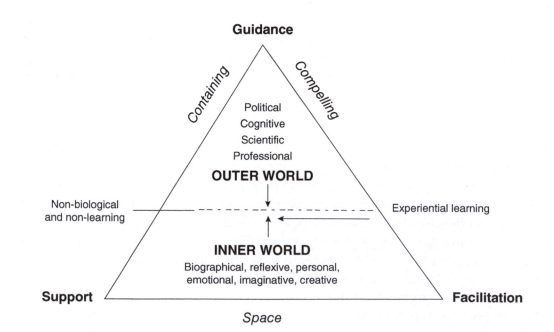

Figure 11.1   Interrelationships between inner and outer worlds of learning and containing and compelling space

Source: Howatson-Jones (2010).

Experiential learning is located at the interface between inner and outer worlds; in other words, your internal world can influence the outer world experiences in which you find yourself and vice versa. For example, consider that you are a spontaneous creative person (inner world). Finding yourself in situations where others are constantly organising you and telling you what you must do and learn can feel constricting and oppressive (outer world). You want to learn to be a professional nurse, so some compromise needs to be reached at the experiential interface between these two worlds. This is where facilitation and support are crucial.

The biographical, personal and emotional dimensions, and reflexive, imaginative and creative responses to these dimensions are influenced by the quality of facilitation and support, and how these qualities may be included or excluded from learning opportunities in spaces that can be somewhat prescriptive. These learning opportunities should link guidance, facilitation and support to help contain anxiety and make learning manageable. Where these are lacking, the interface between inner and outer worlds becomes less fluid, with little chance of critical reflection. The result is non-biographical learning, where nothing is perceived as new, but instead information is just processed with non-awareness and a lack of openness; experiences may be gathered, but nothing learned from them. Consider Scenario 11.5 to make sense of these processes.

Scenario 11.5: Cassie's difficulty with saying no

Cassie was a newly qualified nurse working on a gynaecology ward, which she loved. She had previously been a care worker in a care home before undertaking her nursing programme. Cassie had always been hard working and had completed tasks to a very high standard. Consequently, the nursing home manager had come to rely on Cassie and had frequently asked her to help out when others would not. Cassie had felt flattered to be needed and had complied, even though the extra workload often made her feel stressed and put a strain on family life.

Cassie had undertaken her nursing programme with the blessing of her family. Throughout the programme, she had tried to maintain her family role and study hard. At one stage she did think of quitting because of the strain everything was putting on her. Fortunately, she contacted her personal tutor, who met with her and encouraged Cassie to reflect on what she was doing. This helped Cassie realise that she was taking a passive role, rather than exerting some agency in her life. She did not want to be thought of badly by her family or her colleagues.

In her present role as a newly registered nurse, Cassie decided that she needed some help to overcome the hurdles she was experiencing of having to solve many issues that were unfamiliar. Cassie decided to access clinical supervision, which was

(Continued)

(Continued)

offered by her employer. At the first session her clinical supervisor, Annie, asked Cassie to reflect on her journey from being a care worker to becoming a qualified nurse. Together Cassie and Annie critically examined Cassie's approach to work and noted her tendency to overwork and not be able to say no. Following through the consequences highlighted to Cassie, she realised that she was not learning from what she was experiencing, but instead was trying to conform to others' views. Through Annie's positive guidance Cassie felt confident enough to acknowledge to herself that she was not a bad person, or nurse, if at times she said no. In fact, this might sometimes be the responsible thing to do. Cassie continued to reflect long after leaving the session and was more considered in approaching problems and caring for herself as a result.

Although reflection may be able to address some of the emotional residues of your work, the critical element is vital to avoid becoming ensnared in narcissistic contemplation that does not move you, or your learning, forward. Honestly exploring the line between inner and outer world experience is where awareness of new ideas forms, and is where you can become aware of what you are learning and how to exert some agency within it. Reflecting on the examples given in this chapter and revisiting the NMC's Code (NMC, 2018b), it is interesting to discover that explicit reflection on ensuring quality and maintaining boundaries is woven through the different sections of the Code. You might want to read the section *Practise effectively* (items 6.2, 8.4, 8.7, 9.1–9.4, 11.1–11.3 and 13.3), the section *Practise effectively* (item 15.1) and the section *Promote professionalism and trust* (items 20.6 and 20.9) to reflect on how the NMC's Code (NMC, 2018b) could relate to this scenario.

Chapter summary

Critical reflection is part of being a responsible and accountable practitioner by examining and analysing your practice and learning. As has been noted in this chapter, it requires discipline and systematic thought in order to critically explore what you are doing, and the evidence base of your interpretations and decisions. These aspects can be missed from simple reflection on practice, which often concentrates on emotional elements. The activities in this chapter offer you an opportunity to complete the cycle of connecting feelings, evidence, decisions and actions through critical reflection that takes an analytical view of your practice and development.

Activities and scenarios: Brief outline answers

Activity 11.1 Critical thinking (pages 198–9)

The incident you describe could have been a mistake or something that went particularly well, but you found it important in developing your practice. For example, a mistake could have created feelings of acute anxiety, whereas a compliment could have increased your confidence. What you could do differently would probably relate to improving your knowledge, finding out the facts of the case, seeking help and considering how you use communication. Additional knowledge you might have needed could relate to policies and procedures. The learning that you might take forward is potentially going to relate to communication and decision-making, as well as knowing more about yourself and how you respond to situations. It is important to note that, if the situation were distressing, you might need to reflect on your emotional response first in order to have emotional closure, before you can apply critical reflection to understand aspects of learning in relation to knowledge or skills.

Activity 11.2 Critical reflection on integrating a new member of staff (page 202)

'As the experienced member of staff I could ensure that the new colleague has an induction to the department. I could negotiate expectations clearly, identify sources of information and take time to discuss their experience and knowledge. I could arrange points of contact throughout the day to evaluate, which would allow me to remain informed but give the new person the space to make the necessary decisions. This would reduce situations where they need advice because this might undermine their confidence. I should give constructive feedback to boost her confidence. Maybe I am less of a team player than I think, and could use emotional intelligence by trying to understand the other person's perspective, rather than focusing on how annoying it is to be disturbed. I am used to working autonomously and therefore find it difficult to adjust. I realise that I expect high personal standards and competence from others, but it is unfair to expect this from a colleague who has recently joined the team. I always thought my management style was democratic, but my standards and expectations may be a controlling influence and could limit someone else's development. Outlining organisational and personal needs may help to clarify concerns and I must be aware that feelings of injustice could cloud the relationship with my new colleague, because she has been able to organise flexible working hours.'

'As a new member of staff, I am anxious about getting things right. I have to arrange shifts that are mutually manageable. I am trying to develop my skills through experiencing as much as I can with the support of others, making sure I am doing things correctly. But I am new to this speciality; I feel they think I am a nuisance and that my knowledge is inadequate. I see that the clinical area is busy and I am embarrassed to ask so many questions, but, rather than making a mistake, I want to make sure of what I'm doing. I need to consider the needs of colleagues as well as my own in order to be effective. Discussing expectations and feedback arrangements might help us to find mutually acceptable solutions to my childcare commitments as well as work requirements.'

Activity 11.4 Reflections on Fajid's understanding of young carers (page 205)

Fajid may assume that healthcare and social care are the same thing. He might not understand that there are costs attached to social care. These are financial as well as personal. Social care needs to be paid for. Some people are also reluctant to have strangers caring for them, especially when it involves personal care. It is natural for Kate to want to help her mother. However, taking on too much is likely to impact on her socially and educationally. Equally, if Fajid is not knowledgeable about why children become carers and about available resources, he cannot help Kate's mother to make different choices because she is the adult in this situation. Fajid might want to consider what the nurse's role is in relation to safeguarding children; one might assume that Kate wants to help her mother, but she may feel that she doesn't have a choice. It would be helpful for Fajid to reflect on these issues with his practice supervisor, Simon, to fully understand the breadth and depth of healthcare and social care professionals' roles.

Activity 11.5 Critical thinking (page 205)

The sources of evidence that you might have used are likely to have included the following:

- objective and subjective data to base your assessment on, such as what you found out through communication, what you observed, what you felt, practice policies and theoretical ideas;
- communication and observation are likely to have confirmed whether your interpretation was correct or identified deficits;
- you might have based your decision-making on a protocol, or an assessment of the alternatives and possible consequences, or on intuition or what you had read;
- how you knew it was the right decision would have been through the feedback of others and what you observed the consequences to be.

Activity 11.6 Reflection on Arunda's experience of dealing with pressure (pages 206–7)

Arunda might use the evidence of recognising the significance of vital sign changes to demonstrate her knowledge of physiology. She could also consider the manager's praise as showing she works well under pressure. The manager used Arunda's ability to stay calm under pressure and report changes accurately as evidence that she had embedded knowledge. However, this is only in a narrow field and would not necessarily evaluate all the learning that was required of her in this placement. The practice supervisor is likely to take a broader view and may be using the practice learning assessment criteria to evaluate her learning. She may interpret Arunda's request to go home early as evidence that she does not want to learn. Arunda might feel disadvantaged by her practice supervisor refusing her request, but this is important to learn what it is to be a professional. Although not always convenient, there are times where organisational demands are considered above individual wishes. It is understandable that Arunda would have liked to have time off; she could have requested time off. Planning ahead is part of professional practice; once the duty roster has been completed, any absences result in a staff resource gap. As the department is busy, Arunda should have considered these issues before requesting unscheduled time off. This might be interpreted by the practice supervisor as evidence that Arunda is unable to plan adequately, and that she has insufficient insight and overview of staffing management, which could be expected of a second-year student nurse.

Further reading

Cottrell, S (2011) *Critical Thinking Skills: Developing effective analysis and argument*, 2nd edn. Basingstoke: Palgrave Macmillan.

This book can help you to develop the analysis techniques that are a necessary part of critical reflection.

Metcalfe, M (2006) *Reading Critically at University*. Los Angeles, CA: Sage.

This book can help you to develop understanding of how to review critically sources of information and learning.

Tappen, RM, Weiss, SA and Whitehead, DK (2010) *Essentials of Nursing Leadership and Management*, 5th edn. Philadelphia, PA: FA Davis.

This book can help you to use critical thought in developing in your role, and in developing leadership and management skills.

Glossary

agency how a person makes use of their life resources to develop strategies for change.

analgesia medication that eases pain.

aortic stent insertion a plastic tube that is inserted into the aorta to keep the vessel patent and protect the wall of the vessel.

becoming a process of change that alters a sense of personal identity.

benign MS a mild form of multiple sclerosis (MS) experienced by approximately 10 per cent of sufferers.

catalytic prompting deep exploration and analysis.

cathartic prompting the release of emotion.

clonic descriptive of the jerky movements resulting from muscular spasms.

colonoscopy an investigative procedure involving passing a flexible tube with a camera through the large bowel to visualise the lining and structure.

colostomy where an artificial opening is made and the bowel is brought to the surface to enable the excretion of faeces.

compelling space a space that invites a desire to learn in more meaningful ways.

culture the meanings and understandings held by a group of people that influence the way they think and act.

cyanosed having a lack of oxygen in the tissues, evidenced by a bluish tinge to the lips and fingernails.

ectopic pregnancy a fertilised egg that has lodged in the fallopian tube and is at risk of rupturing the tube as it grows.

empowerment taking personal control.

endoscopy a procedure that visualises the inside of body cavities and tracts using camera technology with a light source and a steerable flexible tube.

epileptic fit a seizure that can manifest itself in a variety of ways and is caused by electrical disruption in the brain.

e-portfolio an electronic portfolio that enables a number of different style documents to be produced, stored and shared.

haemorrhoidectomy removal of haemorrhoids, which are swollen blood vessels usually located in the anal area.

health promotion encouraging people to examine and change their lifestyles to ones that are healthy.

intuition/intuitive knowledge experience-based knowledge.

learning contract a plan of learning objectives agreed between the student and the supervisor.

learning style a preference for particular ways of learning.

life world the history, culture, situations and relationships of an individual.

losing face feeling a loss of respect.

metastases spread of cells and disease (usually cancer) to another part of the body.

multiple sclerosis (MS) incurable neurological condition caused by destruction of the insulation layer surrounding some nerves, which results in disruption of the nerve pathways.

oesophageal gastroduodenoscopy (OGD) a procedure in which a flexible tube with a camera is passed through the oesophagus, stomach and duodenum to visualise the internal lining and structure.

oncology cancer care.

phlebitis inflammation of a vein.

reflection considering and reviewing thinking, actions and circumstances to develop new ideas.

reflective cycle a cyclical structuring of consideration and review of thinking, actions and circumstances to develop new ideas.

reflective framework framing structuring of consideration and review of thinking, actions and circumstances with questions.

reflective practice considering and reviewing the interplay between theory and practice and new ideas.

reflexivity the conscious engagement on the part of the practitioner to being open to examining their own assumptions and influences on situations, and how the cultures and contexts in which they are embedded might be influencing them.

self-concept a perception of who one is and of personal capability.

Skype Skype allows the user to communicate over the internet using voice or video contact so that you can see each other face to face.

socialisation socialisation is a process of developing meaning through interaction and adaptation.

tacit knowledge knowledge that is so deeply embedded that people often forget they have it. It is known to people within a group and does not need explanation within the context of that group, but may be unknown to outsiders.

tonic descriptive of muscle rigidity.

transitional space where a person can consider and try out other ways of being.

trust management unit of NHS healthcare, which may encompass a number of providers and settings.

uterine embolisation deliberate occlusion of the uterine arteries to terminate blood flow.

venepuncture taking a blood sample from a vein.

References

Abrandt Dahlgren, M, Richardson, B and Kalman, H (2004) Redefining the reflective practitioner. In Higgs, J, Richardson, B and Abrandt Dahlgren, M (eds), *Developing Practice Knowledge for Health Professionals*. Edinburgh: Butterworth Heinemann, pp15–34.

Alheit, P and Dausien, B (2007) Lifelong learning and biography: A competitive dynamic between the macro- and the micro-level of education. In West, L, Alheit, P, Andersen Siig, A and Merrill, B (eds), *Using Biographical and Life History Approaches in the Study of Adult and Lifelong Learning: European perspectives*. Frankfurt am Main: Peter Lang, pp57–70.

Andrew, N, Tolson, D and Ferguson, D (2008) Building on Wenger: Communities of practice in nursing. *Nurse Education Today, 28*: 246–52.

Andrew, N, McGuinness, C, Reid, G and Corcoran, T (2009) Greater than the sum of its parts: Transition into the first year of undergraduate nursing. *Nurse Education in Practice, 9*(1): 13–21.

Argyris, C and Schön, D (1978) *Organisational Learning: A theory of action perspective*. Reading, MA: Addison-Wesley.

Armitage, G (2009) The risks of double checking. *Nursing Management, 16*(2): 30–5.

Atkins, S and Murphy, K (1995) Reflective practice. *Nursing Standard, 9*(45): 31–7.

Banks, JA, Au, KH, Ball, AF, Bell, P, Gordon, EW, Gutiérrez, KD, et al. (2007) *Learning in and out of School in Diverse Environments: Life-Long, Life-wide, Life-deep*. Seattle, WA: The LIFE Center (The Learning in Informal and Formal Environments [LIFE] Center).

Barksby, J, Butcher, N and Whysall, A (2015) A new model of reflection for clinical practice. *Nursing Times, 111*(34–5): 21–3.

Bhabha, HK (2004) *The Location of Culture*. Abingdon: Routledge.

Benner, P (1984) *From Novice to Expert: Excellence and power in clinical nursing practice*. Menlo Park, CA: Addison-Wesley.

Bishop, V (2007) *Clinical Supervision in Practice*, 2nd edn. Basingstoke: Palgrave Macmillan.

Boase, C (2008) *Digital Storytelling for Reflection and Engagement: A study of the uses and potential of digital storytelling*. Available at: http://resources.glos.ac.uk/shareddata/dms/766118A3BCD42A03921A19B460003

Bohinc, M and Gradisar, M (2003) Decision-making model for nursing. *Journal of Nursing Administration, 33*(12): 627–9.

Bolton, G (2014) *Reflective Practice: Writing and professional development*, 4th edn. Los Angeles, CA: Sage.

Boud, D and Miller, N (1996) *Working with Experience: Animating learning.* London: Routledge.

Boud, D, Keogh, R and Walker, D (eds) (1985) *Reflection: Turning experience into learning.* London: Kogan Page.

Brechin, A (2000) Introducing critical practice. In Brechin, A, Brown, H and Eby, A (eds), *Critical Practice in Health and Social Care.* London: Sage, pp25–47.

Brockbank, A and McGill, I (2007) *Facilitating Reflective Learning in Higher Education,* 2nd edn. Buckingham: Society for Research into Higher Education/Open University Press.

Brookfield, S (2005) *The Power of Critical Theory for Adult Learning and Teaching.* Maidenhead: Open University Press.

Bulman, C and Schutz, S (eds) (2008) *Reflective Practice in Nursing,* 4th edn. Oxford: Blackwell Science.

Carper, B (1978) Fundamental patterns of knowing in nursing. *Advances in Nursing Science, 1*(1): 13–23.

Cassidy, S (2009) Interpretation of competence in student assessment. *Nursing Standard, 23*(18): 39–46.

Chan, EA and Schwind, JK (2006) Two teachers reflect on acquiring their nursing identity. *Reflective Practice, 7*(3): 303–14.

Chirema, KD (2007) The use of reflective journals in the promotion of reflection and learning in post-registration nursing students. *Nurse Education Today, 27:* 192–202.

Chong, MC (2009) Is reflective practice a useful task for student nurses? *Asian Nursing Research, 3*(3): 111–20.

Coleman, D and Willis, DS (2015) Reflective writing: The student nurse's perspective on reflective writing and poetry writing. *Nurse Education Today, 35*(7): 906–11.

Crabtree, BF (2003) Primary care practices are full of surprises. *Health Care Management Review, 28*(3): 275–83.

Curzon-Hobson, A (2002) A pedagogy of trust in higher learning. *Teaching in Higher Education, 7*(3): 265–76.

Daley, B (2001) Learning in clinical nursing practice. *Holistic Nursing Practice, 16*(1): 43–54.

Dalton, D (2005) Dyslexics should not be discriminated against. *Nursing Standard, 19*(36): 39.

Davidhizar, R and Lonser, G (2003) Storytelling as a teaching technique. *Nurse Educator, 28*(5): 217–21.

Davis, N, Clark, AC, O'Brien, M, Plaice, C, Sumpton, K and Waugh, S (2011) *Learning Skills for Nursing Students.* Exeter: Learning Matters.

Dawber, C (2012) Reflective practice groups for nurses: A consultation liaison psychiatry nursing initiative: Part 1 – the model. *International Journal of Mental Health Nursing, 22*(2): 135–44 de Vries, J and Fiona Timmins, F (2016) Care erosion in hospitals: Problems in reflective nursing practice and the role of cognitive dissonance. *Nurse Education Today, 38*: 5–8.

Department of Health (1997) *The Caldicott Committee Report on the Review of Patient Identifiable Information.* London: HMSO.

Department of Health (2008) *A High Quality Workforce.* London: HMSO.

Department of Health (2009) *The NHS Constitution: Securing the NHS today for generations to come.* London: HMSO.

Department of Health (2012) *Compassion in Practice.* London: DH.

Department of Health (2015) *A Consultation on Updating the NHS Constitution.* Available at: www.gov.uk/government/uploads/system/uploads/attachment_data/file/417637/Update_NHS_Constitution.pdf

Department of Health and NHS Commissioning Board (2012) *Compassion in Practice.* London: Department of Health.

Dix, G and Hughes, SJ (2004) Strategies to help students learn effectively. *Nursing Standard, 18*(32): 39–42.

Dominice, P (2000) *Learning from Ourselves.* San Francisco, CA: Jossey-Bass.

Driscoll, J (2007) *Practising Clinical Supervision: A reflective approach for healthcare professionals,* 2nd revised edn. Edinburgh: Baillière-Tindall.

Ehrmann, G (2005) Managing the aggressive nursing student. *Nurse Educator, 30*(3): 98–100.

Ellis, P (2013) *Evidence-based Practice in Nursing,* 2nd edn. London: Sage.

Ellis, P (2017) *Understanding Ethics for Nursing Students,* 2nd edn. London: Sage.

Ellis, P (2019) *Evidence-based Practice in Nursing,* 3rd edn. London: Sage.

Eraut, M (2001) *Developing Professional Knowledge and Competence,* 2nd edn. London: The Falmer Press.

Esterhuizen, P and Kooyman, A (2001) Empowering moral decision making in nurses. *Nurse Education Today, 21*(8): 640–7.

Falconer, L (2011) Upload and update. *Nursing Standard, 25*(31): 26–7.

Farrell, G (2001) From tall poppies to squashed weeds. *Journal of Advanced Nursing, 35*: 26–33.

Faugier, J and Butterworth, T (1994) Clinical supervision: A position paper. Manchester: University of Manchester.

Field, J (2006) *Lifelong Learning and the New Educational Order,* 2nd edn. Stoke-on-Trent: Trentham Books.

Fischer-Rosenthal, W (2000) Biographical work and biographical structuring in present-day stories. In Chamberlayne, P, Bornat, J and Wengraf, T (eds), *The Turn to Biographical Methods in Social Science: Comparative issues and examples.* London and New York: Routledge, pp109–25.

Francis, R (2010) *Independent Inquiry into Care Provided by Mid Staffordshire NHS Foundation Trust: January 2005–March 2009*, Vol 1. London: HMSO. Available at: www.dh.gov.uk/prod_consum_dh/groups/dh_digitalassets/@dh/@en/@ps/documents/digitalasset/dh_113068.pdf

Francis, R (2013) *Report of the Mid Staffordshire NHS Foundation Trust Public Inquiry: Executive summary.* London: HMSO. Available at: www.midstaffspublicinquiry.com/sites/default/files/report/Executive%20summary.pdf

Freshwater, D (2000) Crosscurrents: Against cultural narration in nursing. *Journal of Advanced Nursing, 32*(2): 481–4.

Freshwater, D, Walsh, E and Esterhuizen, P (2007) Models of effective and reflective teaching and learning for best practice. In Bishop, V (ed.), *Clinical Supervision in Practice: Some questions, answers and guidelines for professionals in health and social care*, 2nd edn. Basingstoke: Palgrave Macmillan

Gerow, L, Conejo, P, Alonzo, A, Davis, N, Rodgers, S and Williams Domian, E (2010) Creating a curtain of protection: Nurses' experiences of grief following patient death. *Journal of Nursing Scholarship, 42*(2): 122–9.

Ghaye, T and Lillyman, S (2010) *Reflection: Principles and practice for healthcare professionals*, 2nd edn. Dinton: Quay Books/Mark Allen.

Gibbs, G (1988) *Learning by Doing: A guide to teaching and learning methods*, RP 391. London: FEU.

Glaze, JE (2001) Stages in coming to terms with reflection: Student advanced nurse practitioners' perceptions of their reflective journeys. *Journal of Advanced Nursing, 37*(3): 263–72.

Hargreaves, J (1997) Using patients: Exploring the ethical dimension of reflective practice in nurse education. *Journal of Advanced Nursing, 25*(2): 223–8.

Hargreaves, J (2004) So how do you feel about that? Assessing reflective practice. *Nurse Education Today, 24*(3): 196–201.

Hawkins, P and Shohet, R (eds) (1989) *Supervision in the Helping Professions.* Philadelphia, PA: Open University Press.

Hawley, MP (2000) Nurse comforting strategies: Perceptions of emergency department patients. *Clinical Nursing Research, 9*(4): 441–59.

Hertz, R (ed.) (1997) *Reflexivity and Voice.* Thousand Oaks, CA: Sage Publications Inc.

Hewitt, O (2014) A survey of experiences of abuse. *Tizard Learning Disability Review, 19*(3): 122–9.

Hinchliff, S, Norman, S and Schober, J (2008) *Nursing Practice and Health Care: A foundation text*, 5th edn. London: Hodder Arnold.

Holmes, J (2005) Notes on mentalizing: Old hat, or new wine? *British Journal of Psychotherapy, 22*(2): 179–97.

Horowitz, SA (2004) The discovery and loss of a 'compelling space': A case study in adapting to a new organisational order. In Huffington, C, Armstrong, D, Halton, W, Hoyle, L and Pooley, J (eds), *Working Below the Surface: The emotional life of contemporary organisations.* London: Karnac, pp151–63.

Horsdal, M (2007) Therapy and narratives of self. In West, L, Alheit, P, Anderson, AS and Merill, B (eds), *Using Biographical and Life History Approaches in the Study of Adult and Lifelong Learning: European perspectives*. Frankfurt am Main: Peter Lang, pp187–203.

Horsdal, M (2012) *Telling Lives: Exploring dimensions of narratives*. London: Routledge.

Howatson-Jones, L (2003) Difficulties in clinical supervision and lifelong learning. *Nursing Standard, 17*(37): 37–41.

Howatson-Jones, L (2010) Exploring the learning of nurses, unpublished PhD thesis, Canterbury Christ Church University/University of Kent, Canterbury.

Howatson-Jones, L (2015a) Ethical aspects of patient assessment dilemmas. In Howatson-Jones, L, Standing, M and Roberts, S (eds), *Patient Assessment and Care Planning in Nursing*, 2nd edn. London: Sage Publications, pp108–20.

Howatson-Jones, L (2015b) Making sense of patient information. In Howatson-Jones, L, Standing, M and Roberts, S (eds), *Patient Assessment and Care Planning in Nursing*, 2nd edn. London: Sage Publications, pp33–50.

Howatson-Jones, L and Thurgate, C (2014) Biographical learning: A process for recovering the soul in nursing. In Formenti, L, West, L and Horsdal, M (eds), *Embodied Narratives: Connecting stories, bodies, cultures and ecologies*. Odense: University Press of Southern Denmark, pp255–73.

Hunt, C and West, L (2007) Salvaging the self in adult learning: Auto/biographical perspectives from teaching and research. Paper presented at the Conference of the ESREA Network on Life History and Biography, Roskilde University, Denmark.

Hurley, J and Linsley, P (2012) *Emotional Intelligence in Health and Social Care*. London: Radcliffe.

Hutchinson, M, Vickers, M, Jackson, D and Wilkes, L (2006) Workplace bullying in nursing: Towards a more critical organisational perspective. *Nursing Inquiry, 13*(2): 118–26.

Iedema, R (2011) Creating safety by strengthening clinicians' capacity for reflexivity. *British Medical Journal Quality and Safety, 20*(suppl 1): i83–6.

Illeris, K (ed.) (2009) *Contemporary Theories of Learning: Learning theorists in their own words*. London: Routledge.

Jacques, D (2000) *Learning in Groups*, 3rd edn. London: Kogan Page.

Jarvis, P (2006) *Towards a Comprehensive Theory of Human Learning. Lifelong Learning and the Learning Society*, Vol 1. London: Routledge.

Jarvis, P (2007) *Globalisation, Lifelong Learning and the Learning Society: Sociological perspectives. Lifelong Learning and the Learning Society*, Vol 2. London: Routledge.

Jarvis, P (2010) *Adult Education and Lifelong Learning: Theory and practice*, 4th edn. New York: Routledge.

Jasper, M (2003) *Beginning Reflective Practice*. Cheltenham: Nelson Thornes.

Johns, C (1995) Framing learning through reflection within Carper's fundamental ways of knowing in nursing. *Journal of Advanced Nursing, 22*: 226–34.

Johns, C (2007) Deep in reflection. *Nursing Standard, 21*(38): 24–5.

Johns, C (2010) *Guided Reflection: A narrative approach to advancing professional practice*, 2nd edn. Chichester: Wiley-Blackwell.

Johns, C (2012) How holistic are we? The role of narrative, storytelling and reflection in the development of holistic practice. *European Journal of Cancer Care, 21*: 561–4.

Johns, C (2013) *Becoming a Reflective Practitioner*, 4th edn. Chichester: John Wiley & Sons, Inc.

Johns, C and Freshwater, D (eds) (2005) *Transforming Nursing Through Reflective Practice*, 2nd edn. Oxford: Blackwell.

Kozlowski, D (2002) Using online learning in a traditional face-to-face environment. *Computers in Nursing, 20*(1): 23–30.

Lachman, VD (2016) Moral resilience: Managing moral distress and moral residue. *MEDSURG Nursing, 25*(2): 121–4.

Lee, NJ (2009) Using group reflection in an action research study. *Nurse Researcher, 16*(1): 30–42.

Lindsay, GM (2006) Constructing a nursing identity: Reflecting on and reconstructing experience. *Reflective Practice, 7*(1): 59–72.

Loughran, JJ (2002). Effective reflective practice: In search of meaning in learning about teaching. *Journal of Teacher Education, 53*(1): 33–43.

Lynch, L, Hancox, K, Happell, B and Parker, J (2008) *Clinical Supervision for Nurses*. Chichester: Wiley-Blackwell.

McCarthy, B, McCarthy, J, Trace, A and Grace, P (2016) Addressing ethical concerns arising in nursing and midwifery students' reflective assignments. *Nursing Ethics*, 1–13.

McCormack, B, Manley, K and Garbett, R (2004) *Practice Development in Nursing*. Oxford: Blackwell Publishing.

McCormack, B, Manley, K and Titchen, A (2013) *Practice Development in Nursing and Healthcare*, 2nd edn. Chichester: Wiley-Blackwell.

Maich, NM, Brown, B and Royle, J (2000) 'Becoming' through reflection and professional portfolios: The voice of growth in nurses. *Reflective Practice, 1*(3): 309–24. Available at: http://ejournals.ebsco.com

Manley, K, Sanders, K, Cardiff, S and Webster, J (2011) Effective workplace culture: The attributes, enabling factors and consequences of a new concept. *International Practice Development Journal, 1*(2): [1].

Manley, K, O'Keefe, H, Jackson, C, Pearce, J and Smith, S (2014) A shared purpose framework to deliver person-centred, safe and effective care: Organisational transformation using practice development methodology. *International Practice Development Journal, 4*(1): [2]. Available at: www.fons.org/Resources/Documents/Journal/Vol4No1/IPDJ_0401_02.pdf

Mason-Whitehead, E and Mason, T (2008) *Study Skills for Nurses*, 2nd edn. Los Angeles, CA: Sage.

Matthews-DeNatale, G (2008) *Digital Story Telling: Tips and resources*. Available at: http://net.educause.edu/ir/library/pdf/ELI08167B.pdf

Milne, D (2009) *Evidence-based Clinical Supervision: Principles and practice*. Oxford: British Psychological Society and Blackwell.

Morton-Cooper, A and Palmer, A (2000) *Mentoring, Preceptorship and Clinical Supervision: A guide to professional support roles in clinical practice*, 2nd edn. Oxford: Blackwell.

Muir, N (2004) Clinical decision-making: Theory and practice. *Nursing Standard, 18*(36): 47–52.

Nåden, D and Eriksson, K (2004) Understanding the importance of values and moral attitudes in nursing care in preserving human dignity. *Nursing Science Quarterly, 17*(1): 86–91.

Nåden, D and Sæteren, B (2006) Cancer patients' perception of being or not being confirmed. *Nursing Ethics, 13*(3): 222–35.

National Society for the Prevention of Cruelty to Children (NSPCC) (2018) Gillick competency and Fraser guidelines: Balancing children's rights with the responsibility to keep them safe from harm. NSPCC Knowledge and Information Services. Available at: https://learning.nspcc.org.uk/media/1541/gillick-competency-factsheet.pdf (accessed 6 January 2019).

Nightingale, F (1969) *Notes on Nursing: What it is and what it is not*. New York: Dover Publications.

Nilsson, B, Nåden, D and Lindström, UÅ (2008) The tune of want in the loneliness melody – loneliness experienced by people with serious mental suffering. *Scandinavian Journal of Caring Sciences, 22*(2): 161–9.

Nursing and Midwifery Council (NMC) (2006) *Clinical Supervision*. London: NMC. Available at: www.nmc-uk.org/aFrameDisplay.aspx?DocumentID=1558

Nursing and Midwifery Council (2012) Social Networking Sites. Available at: www.nmc-uk.org/Nurses-and-midwives/Advice-by-topic/A/Advice/Social-networking-sites

Nursing and Midwifery Council (2017) *Revalidation: How to revalidate with the NMC requirements for renewing your registration*. London: NMC.

Nursing and Midwifery Council (2018a) *Future Nurse: Standards of Proficiency for Registered Nurses*. London: NMC.

Nursing and Midwifery Council (2018b) *The Code: Professional standards of practice and behaviour for nurses and midwives*. London: NMC.

Ohler, J (2008) *Digital Storytelling in the Classroom: New media pathways to literacy, learning and creativity*. Thousand Oaks, CA: Corwin Press.

Ousey, K and Johnson, M (2007) Being a real nurse: Concepts of caring and culture in the clinical areas. *Nurse Education in Practice, 7*(3): 150–5.

Padykula, BM (2017) RN-BS students' reports of their self-care and health-promotion practices in a holistic nursing course. *Journal of Holistic Nursing, 35*(3): 221–46.

Palmer, A, Burns, S and Bulman, C (1994) *Reflective Practice in Nursing: The growth of the professional practitioner.* Oxford: Blackwell Scientific.

Parse, RR (2004) A human becoming teaching–learning model. *Nursing Science Quarterly, 17*(1): 33–5.

Percival, J (2001) Know your enemy. *Nursing Standard, 15*(35): 24–5.

Petty, G (2014) *Teaching Today: A practical guide,* 5th edn. Oxford: Oxford University Press.

Phelan, A, Barlow, C and Iversen, S (2006) Occasioning learning in the workplace: The case of interprofessional peer collaboration. *Journal of Interprofessional Care, 20*(4): 415–24.

Pickersgill, F (2015) It is an enormous privilege to be with people at the end of life. *Nursing Standard, 29* (27): 64–5.

Pierson, W (1998) Reflection and nursing education. *Journal of Advanced Nursing, 27:* 165–70.

Price, B (2008) The intelligent workforce. *Nursing Management, 15*(5): 28–33.

Proctor, B (1986) Supervision: A co-operative exercise in accountability. In Markham, M and Payne, M (eds), *Enabling and Ensuring.* Leicester: National Youth Bureau for Education in Youth and Community Work, pp21–3.

Quality Assurance Agency (QAA) (2014) *The UK Quality Code for Higher Education.* Available at: www.qaa.ac.uk/publications/information-and-guidance/publication?PubID=181#.VVXlUGpwZdh

Ranse, K and Grealish, L (2007) Nursing students' perceptions of learning in the clinical setting of the Dedicated Education Unit. *Journal of Advanced Nursing, 58*(2): 171–9.

Reed, S (2015) *Successful Professional Portfolios for Nursing Students,* 2nd edn. London: Sage/Learning Matters.

Richardson, L (1997) *Fields of Play: Constructing an academic life.* New Brunswick, NJ: Rutgers University Press.

Rogers, C and Freiberg, HJ (1994) *Freedom to Learn,* 3rd edn. New York: Macmillan College.

Rolfe, G (ed.) (2011) *Critical Reflection in Practice: Generating knowledge for caring,* 2nd edn. Basingstoke: Palgrave.

Royal College of Nursing (RCN) (2009) *Legal Advice for RCN Members Using the Internet.* London: RCN. Available at: www.rcn.org.uk/data/assets/pdf_file/0008/272195/003557.pdf

Royal College of Nursing (2011) *Social Networking and Nursing.* Available at: www.rcn.org.uk/newsevents/congress/congress_2011/congress_2011_agenda/9._social_networking_and_nursing

Ruyak, S, Wright, M and Levi, A (2017) Simulation to meet curricular needs in ethics. *Clinical Simulation in Nursing, 13*(3): 121–6.

Scanlan, J and Chernomas, W (1997) Developing the reflective teacher. *Journal of Advanced Nursing, 25*(6): 1138–43.

Schmidt, NA (2008) Guided imagery as internally orientated self-care: A nursing case. *Self-care, Dependent-care and Nursing, 16*(1): 41–8.

Schön, D (1987) *Educating the Reflective Practitioner: Toward a new design for teaching and learning in the professions.* San Francisco, CA: Jossey-Bass.

Schön, D (1991) *The Reflective Practitioner: How professionals think in action.* Farnham: Arena, Ashgate.

Sennett, R (2008) *The Craftsman.* London: Allen Lane/Penguin Books.

Smith, A and Jack, K (2005) Reflective practice: A meaningful task for students. *Nursing Standard, 19*(26): 33–7.

Standing, M (2017) *Clinical Judgement and Decision-making for Nursing Students,* 3rd edn. London: Sage.

Stephenson, S and Holm, D (1994) Reflection: A student's perspective. In Palmer, A, Burns, S and Bulman, C (eds), *Reflective Practice in Nursing: The growth of the professional practitioner.* Oxford: Blackwell Science Publishing, p137.

Sully, P and Dallas, J (2010) *Essential Communication Skills for Nursing and Midwifery,* 2nd edn. Edinburgh: Elsevier Mosby.

Tappen, RM, Weiss, SA and Whitehead, DK (2010) *Essentials of Nursing Leadership and Management,* 5th edn. Philadelphia, PA: FA Davis.

Taylor, B (2010) *Reflective Practice for Healthcare Professionals,* 3rd edn. Maidenhead: Open University Press.

Thompson, C and Dowding, D (eds) (2002) *Clinical Decision-making and Judgement in Nursing.* Edinburgh: Churchill Livingstone.

Thorndycraft, B and McCabe, J (2008) The challenge of working with staff groups in the caring professions: The importance of the 'Team Development and Reflective Practice Group'. *British Journal of Psychotherapy, 24*(2): 167–82.

Titchen, A and McGinley, M, with McCormack, B (2004) Blending self-knowledge and professional knowledge. In Higgs, J, Richardson, B and Abrandt Dahlgren, M (eds), *Developing Practice Knowledge for Health Professionals.* Edinburgh: Butterworth Heinemann, pp107–26.

Turkel, MC, Watson, J and Giovannoni, J (2018) Caring science or science of caring. *Nursing Science Quarterly, 31*(1): 66–7.

United Kingdom Central Council (UKCC) for Nursing, Midwifery and Health Visiting (1994) *The Future of Professional Practice: The Council's standard for education and practice following registration.* London: UKCC.

van Boven, L, White, K, Kamada, A and Gilovich, T (2003) Intuitions about situational correction in self and others. *Journal of Personality and Social Psychology, 85*(2): 249–58.

van Ooijen, E (2013) *Clinical Supervision Made Easy,* 2nd edn. Monmouth: PCCS Books.

Watson, J (1988) *Nursing: Human Science and Human Care: A theory of nursing.* New York: National League for Nursing.

Watson, J (2008) *Nursing: The Philosophy and Science of Caring,* revised edn. Boulder, CO: University Press of Colorado.

West, L (2001) *Doctors on the Edge: General practitioners' health and learning in the inner city.* London: Free Associates Books.

West, L, Alheit, P, Anderson, AS and Merill, B (eds) (2007) *Using Biographical and Life History Approaches in the Study of Adult and Lifelong Learning: European perspectives.* Frankfurt am Main: Peter Lang.

Willis, P, Lord (2015) *Raising the Bar. Shape of Caring: A review of the future education and training of registered nurses and care assistants.* HEE in association with the NMC. Available at: http://hee.nhs.uk/2015/03/12/the-shape-of-caring-review-report-published

Wiman, E and Wikblad, K (2004) Caring and uncaring encounters in nursing in an emergency department. *Journal of Clinical Nursing, 13*(4): 422–9.

Winnicott, DW (1965) *The Maturational Processes and the Facilitating Environment: Studies in the theory of emotional development.* London: Karnac and the Institute of Psycho-Analysis.

Xu, Y and Davidhizar, R (2005) Intercultural communication in nursing education: When Asian students and American faculty converge. *Journal of Nursing Education, 44*(5): 209–15.

Zander, PE (2007) Ways of knowing in nursing: The historical evolution of a concept. *Journal of Theory Construction and Testing, 11*(1): 7–11.

Index

Note: Page references in **bold** refer to the Glossary, those in *italic* to figures and tables.